600 AROMATHERAPY RECIPES

for

Beauty, Healthy & Home

600 AROMATHERAPY RECIPES

for

Beauty, Healthy & Home

by

Beth Jones

Before reading or following any of the recipes in this book, it is very important to familiarize yourself with the safety guidelines outlined in Chapter 9. Essential oils are highly concentrated liquids and can be harmful if used incorrectly. All safety guidelines must be strictly followed. The author is not responsible for any mishandling or negligence by the user while using any of the recipes in this book. All oils must be allergy tested before use and the onus is on the user to carry out allergy testing. The safety guidelines, outlined in Chapter 9, are not a complete safety reference for the use of essential oils, if in doubt, a doctor or physician must be consulted regarding any health issues.

First published July 2014

ISBN-13: 978-1500770297
ISBN-10: 1500770299

Other Books by Beth Jones
1,001 Ways to Use Essential Oils – Including 61 Essential Oils

Table of Contents

Introduction

Part One

Part Two

Part Three

11 Aromatherapy for Health 120

Part Four

12   Aromatherapy for the Home   **209**

Introduction

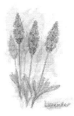

Aromatherapy is the use of essential oils, extracted from various parts of aromatic plants and trees, to promote health of the body and serenity of mind. It is considered a holistic therapy, which makes use of the various properties of these oils, incorporating them into various forms of treatment, aimed at restoring and maintaining health.

Like all holistic therapies, aromatherapy seeks to strengthen the body's own innate self-healing ability, aiming to restore balance, both physically and psychologically. It views disease or disorder as the result of an imbalance in the body or mind, and strives to correct this. This imbalance usually occurs when a person moves further away from a more 'natural' way of living, which may involve eating the wrong foods, lack of exercise or allowing the mind to become preoccupied with negative thoughts. Making appropriate lifestyle changes is an important part of an aromatherapy treatment, and will greatly compliment the properties of essential oils, helping to speed healing.

Aromatherapy treatments may take the form of;

❖   An aromatherapy massage, which is not only the most cost effective and safest way of introducing oils to the body, but it also includes the values of the actual massage therapy itself, and the importance of therapeutic touch.
❖   The oils may also be incorporated into a bath,
❖   Used on a compress.
❖   Used as inhalations.
❖   They can be used in an oil burner, which can produce a wonderful fragrant atmosphere in a room.
❖   They are a valuable addition to any beauty routine being used in both the care of skin and hair, and can make highly pleasant perfumes when applied to the skin.

These oils can expel their physical and psychological benefits, regardless of what form of treatment is used, as their effects are exerted both by the absorption of minute quantities of the oil through the skin, and inhalation of the evaporated oil into the lungs from the air.

Although each essential oil will have individual properties and characteristics of its own, they are all antiseptic and most are also endowed with antiviral or anti-inflammatory properties. They promote natural healing by stimulating and reinforcing the body's' own mechanisms, and exert an influence over the central nervous system. Some will help others stimulate, while some have the ability to normalize or balance the system. Certain oils have the remarkable ability to stimulate the growth and regeneration of skin cells, useful both in healing and rejuvenation. They aim to strengthen the immune system, and although certain oils have the ability to exert their influence very strongly in all of the above conditions, all essential oils have these properties to some extent, as well as other individual characteristics.

Aromatherapy is therefore a valuable form of holistic treatment, working to free the body's own innate healing force, thereby allowing balance to be restored, a state of equilibrium in which disease or disorder cannot manifest. It is a natural, gentle therapy, which once practiced in a controlled and professional manner, can do much to re-balance the body and mind. A most fascinating aspect of aromatherapy is the influence of aroma on the mind and emotions, due to the mind-body link. Any alteration in the emotional state will often bring about a beneficial change in the physical body as well, making aromatherapy a valuable treatment for the whole person.

1
About Essential Oils

Essential oils are the basic materials of the aromatherapist, and although sometimes referred to as essences, this description is incorrect, as the essence is what is actually produced by the plant, becoming known as an essential oil only after distillation. This process causes certain chemical changes to take place in the various constituents of the essence, but the therapeutic value is not harmed and even seems to be enhanced. In the same vein, although the term 'essential oils' is used loosely to describe all the oils used in Aromatherapy, those obtained by methods other than distillation should not, strictly speaking, be so called. The citrus oils, for example, extracted by simple pressure, are still in the form of the simple essence when we use them, whereas the floral oils of Jasmine, Neroli and Rose, obtained by enfleurage, should rightly be classed as Absolutes. However the term essential oil is generally used to describe these odoriferous, volatile liquid components of plants, which accumulate in specialized cells in specific parts of the plant, seeds, leaves, flowers, bark, roots or resin etc.

The proportion of essence contained in a plant will vary a great deal from species to species, which accounts in part for the varying prices of essential oils, the amounts also varying according to the growing conditions and the time of harvesting. Sometimes different oils, with different therapeutic properties, can be extracted from different parts of the same plant.

The orange tree, for example, produces Neroli from the blossom, Petitgrain from the leaves and Orange oil from the skin of the fruit.

Essential oils are said to be produced by the plant for its own survival, to repel predators and protect itself from disease. They are said to influence fertilization of the plant by attracting pollinating insects, and in this way could be likened to the pheromones secreted by humans and animals. Another line of thought is that they are actually the hormones of the plant, and influence growth and production in the plant itself, in much the same way as our hormones influence us. This seems realistic as the quantity of hormones produced during the whole lifetime of an individual could quite easily be compared to that produced by a single plant in its lifetime.

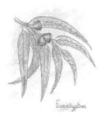

Due to this relationship, essential oils can be used to balance the human body, through their effects on our hormones, either duplicating or potentiating their effects, whatever is required to restore harmony. They have the added benefit of being organic substances which blend in well with the body, unlike inorganic substances or drugs which may be liable to cause quite severe side-effects.

Being organic, they are living substances and therefore contain life force, as evidenced by *Kirlian Photography*, and are said to be the source of the life force in the plant itself, which can greatly compliment the life force of the human body. Just as the human body is influenced by diet, lifestyle, surroundings, climate and even time of day, the quality of an essential oil is similarly influenced. Soil conditions, climate, altitude and the time of harvesting can all influence quality. Certain plants need to be picked at a certain time of day, where concentration of the oil in the plant is at its highest, or when the chemical composition is in the required state, which can also change according to the time of day or season.

It is important to complete the process of harvesting as quickly as possible and to obtain oil that has been produced by plants living in their natural environment. These factors will ensure the minimum loss of oil through evaporation, and also ensure that the oil has been produced from plants grown in a soil and climate best suited to the quality of the plant and therefore its oil.

When buying from a supplier, it is important that they have a reputable name in the trade. A good safeguard is to buy from someone who can provide the following information;

❖ The country or region of origin
❖ The botanical name of the plant
❖ The part of the plant used
❖ The method of extraction
❖ Whether the plant is wild or organically grown

Unlike ordinary oils, such as corn or sunflower, the majority of essential oils have the consistency of water, and are not greasy. They dissolve easily in ordinary fatty oils such as avocado or sweet almond oil. They also dissolve easily in wax products, such as melted beeswax or jojoba. It is important to note that they do not dissolve in water. They will ignite easily and can be quite varied in their depth and intensity of color. Some are almost colorless, or of pastel shades, while others are deeply pigmented. Where colors can omit certain healing vibrations, oils of the same color will possess the same therapeutic value. Blue, for example, is cooling, calming and relaxing. Chamomile oil which has a blue tint, is used to reduce inflammation, and has a calming, soothing effect on the body and mind.

Essential oils promote natural healing by stimulating and reinforcing the body's own mechanisms. Where all oils are antiseptic, some also contain one or more of the following properties;

- anti-sudorific
- anti-viral
- anti-bacterial
- anti-inflammatory
- anti-rheumatic
- anti-spasmodic
- calming
- relaxing
- carminative
- cicatrisant
- expectorant
- sedative
- laxative
- diuretic
- anti-depressant
- depurative

Unlike chemical antiseptics, most essential oils, when used correctly, are harmless to the body tissues, while at the same time being powerful aggressors towards germs and wound healing. Chamomile, among others, is credited with the ability to stimulate the production of white blood cells which help in our fight against disease, while Lavender has the remarkable ability to stimulate the regeneration of skin cells helping in the healing of burns, scar tissue, wounds and ulcers. Essential oils also act on the nervous system, Chamomile and Lavender having a relaxing effect, while Rosemary and Basil a more stimulating effect. Certain oils actually have the ability to normalize, regardless of the problem, for example, Bergamot and Geranium have both sedating or stimulating properties according to the specific needs of the individual.

On the whole essential oils act by re-balancing the body, mind and emotions through their absorption into the body through the skin, and through the tiny air sacs of the lungs after inhalation.

The chemistry of essential oils is complex with one single oil potentially consisting of hundreds of different components. These components are usually grouped into the following main categories;

> **Acids** – anti-inflammatory
> **Alcohols** – antiseptic, anti-viral, anti-fungal, energizing, uplifting.
> **Aldehydes** – anti-inflammatory, anti-fungal, disinfectant, uplifting, sedative.
> **Coumarins** – sedative, uplifting, hypotensive.
> **Ethers** – sedative, calming, anti-spasmodic, balancing, soothing.
> **Esters** – balancing, soothing, calming, relaxing, anti-inflammatory.
> **Ketones** – stimulating, warming.
> **Lactones** – anti-inflammatory, expectorant.
> **Monoterpenes** – stimulating, warming, decongestant, expectorant, anti-viral.
> **Oxides** – antiseptic, expectorant, stimulating.
> **Phenols** – stimulating, anti-infectious, anti-spasmodic, anti-bacterial.
> **Sesquiterpenes** – anti-inflammatory, anti-allergy, antiseptic, calming.
> **Terpenes** – anti-infectious, stimulating, tonic, antiseptic, anti-inflammatory, anti-viral.

It is the unique combination of chemicals found in each plant that gives it its characteristic perfume and therapeutic properties. The combination of chemicals contained in each oil act synergistically, balancing and affecting each other's properties in such a way as to bring about a beneficial change in the physical or mental body. This change is able to take place without the risk of certain side effects, which are so often produced when chemists try to isolate a single 'active ingredient' from the plant essence in the treatment of a specific disorder.

The composition of essential oils will differ depending upon which part of the plant the oil is contained within, for example, those from flowers have a much more complicated composition than those from leaves. In their natural 'mixed state', essential oils are otherwise known as Terpenoids, because terpenes are present in the greatest quantity. In this 'whole state' the oil is infinitely superior to any man-made alternative, with certain molecules in the oil reinforcing the action of the whole.

All essential oils have their own individual characteristics and properties. While certain oils can be used alone to treat a number of different disorders, these oils often work best when mixed together as they complement and enhance each other's properties in much the same way as a single oil will work best as a 'whole' rather than when it is divided into it constituents parts.

2
How Aromatherapy Works: The Body

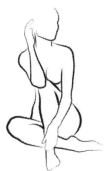

Aromatherapy works by influencing at least 2 levels simultaneously, the physical and emotional, and as all levels interrelate, the spiritual aspect of the individual will also be affected, although in a much more subtle way. The established effects of essential oils on the human organism can therefore be divided into 2 kinds, physiological and psychological, with the former acting directly on the physical body, and the latter acting, via the sense of smell, on the mind, which in turn may also cause a physiological effect.

Although these two levels may be perceived as separate, it would be difficult to explain how essential oils can affect one specific level, without influencing the other, as it is the actual ability of aromatherapy to treat the 'whole' individual that makes it such as effective and recommended form of treatment.

Physiological effects can be further divided into two types;

- ➢ Those which act via the nervous system, and to a small extent, the endocrine system
- ➢ Those which act directly on an organ or tissue of the body itself.

Where these two effects can be described as being quite separate, it is almost certain that they may occur simultaneously, especially when appropriate oils are used.

The skin and the lungs are both vital to aromatherapy, as these are the two routes by which essential oils enter the body. The skin is the body's largest organ, which is primarily concerned with the elimination of waste products, which result from everyday bodily processes. It can be described as being semi-permeable, as it completely surrounds the body, acting as a protective covering, allowing certain substances to pass through, while preventing others from gaining access.

What determines the ability of any substance to be able to pass through the skin, or not, is the size of the molecules from which it is made up. Water and watery substances cannot be absorbed into small enough, can certainly gain access. Essential oils have very fine aromatic molecules, and can be absorbed through the skin quite easily.

It is thought that essential oils pass through the hair follicles, which contain sebum, an oily liquid with which the essential oils have a particular affinity, and from here, diffuse into the fine blood capillaries which lie just under the surface of the skin. Alternatively, they are taken up by the lymph and interstitial fluid to be carried to other parts of the body.

Aromatherapy massage offers the safest and most effective way of introducing essential oils into the body, and when diluted in a suitable carrier oil, the ability of essential oils to be absorbed through the skin is further enhanced.

If the skin is healthy, it may take only a few minutes for the initial absorption of the essential oils to take place, but it will take much longer if the skin is congested, either from the inside with toxins, or from the outside with dirt.

In this regard, the state of the skin in general will play an important part in determining how long it will take for the essential oil treatments to have significant effect. This does not mean, however, that aromatherapy would be of no benefit to people with congested skins, it would in fact be a most beneficial form of treatment under these circumstances, as it would begin the re-balancing process. In these cases an appropriate change in lifestyle could considerably increase the value of treatments and the speed of healing, especially with regard to sufficient fresh air and exercise, coupled with an improvement in the overall diet. These changes would greatly reduce the toxic elements in the blood, and would allow the other organs of elimination, the kidneys and colon, to carry out their work efficiently, without having to rely on the skin to remove any excess waste, putting it under unnecessary strain. Also the 'cleaner' condition of the blood itself will facilitate the smooth and more efficient passage of essential oils throughout the body.

A large amount of fatty tissue, water retention, and poor circulation will also impede the absorption and passage of essential oils in the body, so it really depends on the condition of each individual as to the actual absorption time, which can vary from as little as 1 hour in some people, to 24 hours in others. The lymph, even more so than the blood, will not carry the oils efficiently if it is congested. Unlike the blood, it is not assisted to any great extent in its flow and tends to become stagnant when congested. This system, however, can be greatly improved by regular massage especially when combined with appropriate oils, and a suitable change in diet. It is important to remember that although the oils may be absorbed through the skin in a matter of minutes, in some cases, their journey is far from over, and may take some time before they actually reach their designated organs, where they begin to influence their effects.

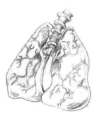 The aromatic molecules of essential oils can also enter the body by way of the lungs. When these molecules are inhaled, they eventually reach the tiny air sacs of the lungs, from where they diffuse into the tiny blood capillaries. In this way, the oils will eventually enter the main blood vessels and enter the body as gases, influencing their effect. Although absorption via the lungs can be a very beneficial means of getting essential oils into the body, it does not offer the advantages of massage. Apart from the benefits of therapeutic touch during massage, the oils can be applied generally, over the whole body in a wider area, thus reaching their designated organs much quicker. It is also possible to treat a local area directly, by applying the oil over such an area, or by guiding the oil to exactly where it is needed.

It should also be remembered that certain emotions can become stored in the body as physical tensions, and the gradual breaking down and releasing of these tensions during massage, will give rise to the subsequent release of these emotions, ones that may have been stored in the body for some time. Inhalation of essential oils does not offer this advantage, unless appropriate oils are used over a long period of time. Massage however, can produce this result on its own, and when combined with the use of appropriate essential oils the results can be nothing short of amazing.

Once they have entered the bloodstream, essential oils diffuse from the blood and/or lymph, and enter the various organs and tissues of the body via the extracellular fluid. Appropriate oils are taken up and held by the different parts of the body that require them. This ability of the body to 'pick and choose', is said to be the result of the actual synergistic action of the individual oils themselves. This phenomenon is probably coupled with the body's own innate ability to know exactly what each organ and tissue of the body needs in order to regain and maintain a healthy balance.

3

Action of Aromatherapy on the Individual Body System

The Lymphatic System

The lymphatic system is not only responsible for the removal of toxic wastes from all parts of the body, but it is also involved in the absorption of fats from the intestines. This important system, along with the adrenal glands and spleen, plays an important part in the immune response, which is the body's attempt to defend itself against disease.

Essential oils, by stimulating the production of white blood cells and other organs involved in the immune response, not only strengthen the body's stand against infection, but through their bactericidal, antiviral and fungicidal properties, they can actually support the body directly by opposing micro-organisms that threaten its defense.

➢ Lavender, Bergamot, Eucalyptus and Rosemary not only stimulate the workings of the body's lymphatic system, but also act directly against a wide range of bacteria and viruses.

➢ The adrenal glands, also important in the immune response, are supported by the oils of Rosemary and Geranium, which also act as a general stimulant to the immune system as a whole.

➢ Cajeput, Niaouli and Tea Tree combine bactericidal, antiviral and fungicidal properties with a particularly powerful stimulant action on the organs involved in the immune response.

➢ Although most essential oils possess the above properties to some degree, Lavender, Bergamot, Lemon and Tea Tree are the ones which have the most marked effects in these regards.

➢ The spleen, another organ involved with the immune response, is supported by all the actions of Black Pepper and Lavender, the former also being implicated as a good oil for encouraging a more efficient drainage of lymph, to be used alternatively with Rosemary, if treatment is to be continued over a long period.

> When essential oils and massage are combined, a more efficient drainage of lymph is encouraged. Fennel, Geranium, Juniper, Rosemary and Black Pepper being of particular importance here, and as several of these oils are also diuretic in action, they will encourage the excretion of such wastes via the kidneys.

Massage offers the most effective therapy for use on the lymphatic system, encouraging lymph circulation and the drainage of cells through the body, thus preventing a buildup of toxins in the tissues, which can lead to edema, adhesions or deposits around the muscles and joints, leading to pain, stiffness and loss of mobility, and cellulitis.

The value of essential oils in relaxing and balancing a person, mentally and emotionally, must not be forgotten. During an aromatherapy massage the person will also be inhaling the aroma of the oils and will be influenced by them in this way too. There is a strong connection between the emotional field and the body's immune system, so it is always important to blend the oils accordingly, where a person's immune system may be depressed due to an emotional imbalance. It is a well known fact that the adrenal glands can become exhausted due to prolonged or acute periods of stress, so oils that not only support and strengthen the immune response, but also instill deep relaxation, can be of extreme value in treating this system, Lavender being an excellent example.

The Nervous System

The action of essential oils, and also massage, on the various activities of the nervous system form a major part of aromatherapy, as this system more than any other is strongly involved in the mind-body link. As a result, anything that will benefit this system will have a pronounced effect on the organism as a whole.

> Oils in general, which produce a beneficial effect on the nervous system, include Chamomile, Clary Sage, Juniper, Lavender, Marjoram, Melissa and Rosemary.
> Bergamot, Chamomile, Lavender and Marjoram have analgesic, antispasmodic and sedative properties, helping to relieve pain, promote a calming effect, and reduce over-activity of the nervous system.
> Eucalyptus, Peppermint and Rosemary are both analgesic and antispasmodic, helping to relieve pain and calm nerves which trigger muscle activity, but they are not sedative.
> Because of the effects produced by the above oils on this system, they are most commonly the ones used in aromatherapy, especially where there is pain or spasm in the voluntary muscles or internal organs.

- Oils which combine both sedative and antispasmodic effects are Clary Sage, Cypress, Juniper, Melissa, Neroli, Rose and Sandalwood.
- Neroli oil has a marked effect on the autonomic nerves which govern the intestines, and Sandalwood acting particularly on the nerves of the bronchial passages, useful for calming down a cough caused by nervous reflex action.
- Although most oils can be described as either stimulating or sedative, each oil can in fact possess both qualities, depending on the amount of the particular oil used. Peppermint, for example, has been found to be stupefying in large doses and stimulating when used in only small amounts.
- Some oils such as Bergamot and Geranium, have a normalizing effect, and will stimulate or sedate, depending on the needs of the individual.
- Rosemary produces a marked stimulant effect on the central nervous system and is of particular value where there is loss or reduction of function in either sensory or motor nerves. It is a powerful brain stimulant and helps to improve memory and aids concentration, clearing and sharpening the mind generally.

When massage is combined with appropriate oils, the effects on the nervous system can be quite pronounced. The lightest of strokes can produce a strong relaxation effect through the body as a whole, especially when performed on the more sensitive parts of the body such as the face, hands or feet, areas more liberally supplied with nerve endings. The body will respond to therapeutic touch, and where a person may be lethargic or need energizing, firmer, more brisk strokes could be used. Alternatively, slower, smoother strokes could be used on someone who was perhaps over-anxious and stressed, with appropriate oils to instill calm and deep relaxation.

Essentially, aromatherapy massage can do much to balance the autonomic nervous system, with particular regard to the sympathetic system, which so often predominates in the individual, due to the stressful times in which we live.

The Digestive System

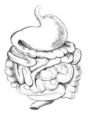 The antispasmodic, calmative and digestive actions of essences are well known, herbs and spices having long been used in foods to encourage the flow of digestive juices, and discourage stomach spasms and flatulence. These properties are entirely due to the essential oils that such herbs and spices contain.

The initial stage of digestion is olfaction, or smell, the very aroma of food stimulating the secretion of digestive juices. In fact, taste plays quite a small part, as our taste buds can only perceive four basic flavors, so the greater part of what we commonly call the 'taste' of food, is actually its 'smell', evidenced by the fact that food loses its taste when our nose is blocked. So it would appear that the digestive action of essential oils is primarily due to their effect via the sense of olfaction.

- ➤ Camphor, Cinnamon, Fennel, Marjoram and Rosemary are useful in constipation, flatulence and lack of intestinal tone, exerting these effects by strengthening peristalsis, which also produces a relatively mild laxative effect.
- ➤ The opposite effect, that of reducing smooth muscle spasm or promoting antispasmodic action is observed in a large number of essences such as Bergamot, Lavender, Cypress and Neroli.
- ➤ Thyme oil can counteract adrenalin spasm, while Melissa and Sage are among those which reduce acetylcholine spasm.
- ➤ Clove oil counteracts stomach acidity by effectively raising the PH of gastric juice, and as this is due to its engerol content, similar effects may be observed with Cinnamon Leaf and Black Pepper.
- ➤ The action of Clary, Clove, Fennel, Peppermint, Rose, and Thyme is considered to be direct, while that of Melissa and Sage are known to occur through the nervous system.

Essential oils should never be taken orally, but aromatherapy massage and compresses applied directly over the abdomen, offer effective ways of introducing oils into the digestive system. Massage can be given along each side of the spine, from where the nerves, which influence this system, arise. It can also be applied directly over the abdomen, and in this way the digestive system can also benefit from the mechanical effect of the massage itself, as well the reflex effect and the properties of the essential oils used in the massage. The reflex effect of the massage alone is very noticeable, and the lightest touch on the abdomen will stimulate the peristaltic action of the intestines, helping to move the products for digestion along the tract and assist in the elimination of wastes from the colon.

Massage, through its effect on the nervous system, will also cause an increase in the secretions of the small intestine and its associated glands, thereby aiding the digestion of food. Through this reflex effect, the small arteries in the abdomen dilate, thus increasing the supply of blood in this area and facilitating a more efficient absorption of food elements through the intestines, as well as promoting the absorption and passage of the essential oils used. The mechanical effect of the massage is confined to the large intestine, where clockwise massage movements can physically assist in the passage and final elimination of waste from the colon, presenting another positive aid to elimination and helping to prevent constipation.

The Cardiovascular System

The cardiovascular system comprises of the heart and blood vessels.

- ➤ The heart muscle can actually be strengthened by oils of Garlic, Borneol, Lavender, Marjoram, Peppermint, Rosemary and Geranium, these oils often being described as tonics.
- ➤ Lavender, Melissa, Neroli and Ylang Ylang are recommended for palpitations and other disorders of the heart which arise due to anxiety or nerves.
- ➤ Calamus is another oil which appears to have an antispasmodic effect on the heart muscle, and it also has the ability to reduce blood pressure, probably due to its similar effect on the blood vessel walls.
- ➤ In fact, most oils that have an antispasmodic effect on the heart, such as the latter oils mentioned, will produce this action on the blood vessel walls, and therefore encourage the blood pressure within the vessels to drop. This action generally takes place via the autonomic nervous system.
- ➤ The opposite effect can also be produced by the use of certain stimulant oils, thereby causing a rise in blood pressure due to contraction of the blood vessel walls.
- ➤ Camphor is one particular oil that has the ability to increase blood pressure, also acting as a cardiac stimulant. Other stimulant oils can also produce the same effects, Hyssop, Rosemary, Sage, Juniper, Cinnamon and Benzoin for example.
- ➤ Hyssop oil, however, could be best described as producing a tonic effect on this system as it can cause an increase in blood pressure, followed by a decrease.
- ➤ Rosemary oil can be useful in the treatment of atherosclerosis, as it helps to lower cholesterol levels in the blood, helping to prevent the buildup of fatty substances on the inside of the blood vessel walls.

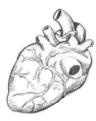 The effects of massage on the circulation are well established. By assisting and encouraging the flow of blood around the body, massage can greatly reduce the pressure that the heart must exert to keep the blood flowing, particularly venous blood. This effect is produced by the mechanical effect of massage, but the reflex effect, or the body's response through the nervous system, will cause the small arteries to dilate, resulting in a greater volume of blood entering the tissues. This will further reduce the pressure on the heart, essentially promoting a reduction in blood pressure, and therefore also taking strain off the blood vessels themselves, improving their condition.

Massage can be particularly beneficial to this system when it is applied over the dorsal area, guiding the essential oils to the target organs. The oils can also be applied in the form of a compress, which can be placed directly over the heart area. Baths and inhalations are also a means by which essential oils can be introduced into the blood circulation, and therefore the other organs of the body.

The Endocrine System

Essential oils can benefit the endocrine system in two different ways. Some oils contain plant hormones, known as phytohormones, which are similar in action to our own, and act within the human body in a similar manner, thereby reinforcing or replacing the effects of certain hormones which may be lacking. Fennel, for example, contains a plant estrogen, and can be used beneficially in menopausal and pre menstrual problems, also helping to stimulate the production of breast milk.

The other way in which essential oils can affect the endocrine system is by actually stimulating the various glands themselves, thereby stimulating the secretion of hormones from these glands or balancing hormone production. The health of the body being dependant on the correct output of hormones from each gland.

> Garlic, for example, helps to balance thyroid secretions, proving particularly beneficial when this gland is under active.
> Basil, Geranium, Pine, Rosemary and Sage are said to stimulate the adrenal cortex, with Geranium being known as the balancer of hormone production in general.
> Eucalyptus and Juniper appear to assist in the reduction of excessive blood sugar levels, with Geranium again, acting as a balancer in this regard.
> As well as Fennel, essential oils such as Chamomile, Clary Sage, Cypress, Jasmine, Lavender and particularly Rose, affect the reproductive system and are useful for rebalancing this system when problems occur.

The pronounced effect of aromatic oils on the emotions, the nervous system, their aphrodisiac affect, and their effect on the body in general, would seem to indicate endocrine influence, an influence which not only exerts its effects via the glands themselves, the nervous system and a mimicking of our own hormones, but also it would appear on a more subtle level, through the sense of smell. The olfactory area of the brain connects with the hypothalamus, a vital structure which controls the entire hormonal system through its influence on the pituitary gland. The hypothalamus also exerts an influence over the autonomic nervous system, and is the means by which the endocrine system interrelates with this part of the nervous system and vice versa.

The Respiratory System

The antiseptic, antispasmodic and expectorant action of essential oils is of extreme value in treating disorders of the respiratory system.

> For general use on this system, Bergamot, Cinnamon and Eucalyptus appear to be the most valuable. The antiseptic qualities of essential oils make them an ideal means of treating and preventing all types of respiratory infections.

> Bergamot, Garlic, Camphor and Eucalyptus were found to be most effective against various infections such as pneumonia, diphtheria and influenza.

> For general use against flu viruses, Cinnamon, Eucalyptus and Black Pepper are most useful. These oils have also been proved valuable by protecting a healthy individual during flu and other epidemics, helping to prevent infection by air-borne bacteria.

> Clary Sage, Fennel, Peppermint, Rose and Thyme, all show an antispasmodic effect on smooth muscle, an effect which is considered to be direct, and are valuable in treating any disorder due to muscular spasm of the air passages, with resultant congestion.

> The choice of oils will depend on many factors; whether or not infection is present, whether the condition is due to an allergic response, or whether emotional factors are involved – stress and anxiety often being the initial cause of such conditions.

> Chamomile is useful where allergies may be involved.

> Bergamot, Lavender and Eucalyptus are good for chest infections, and these antiseptic oils, as well as Chamomile, Peppermint, Basil and Neroli are all antispasmodic oils, the latter being of particular help if the disorder is due to an emotional problem.

> Camphor oil is a general respiratory stimulant and increases both the rate and amplitude of respiration.

> Eucalyptus, Lemon and Frankincense were found to be particularly beneficial for their expectorant action.

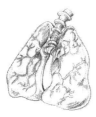 Essential oils for respiratory complaints may be given by inhalations, steam inhalations, spinal massage, especially to the cervical and dorsal area, or massage of the thoracic area. Compresses applied to these areas can also be of extreme value. If an asthma sufferer is experiencing a bad attack, steam inhalation should be avoided, as the heat of the latter will increase any inflammation of the mucus membranes and make the congestion even worse.

It should be remembered that this system is one of the means by which essential oils gain access to the body, enabling them to influence their effects. The nose forms the first part of the respiratory system, through which essential oils, taken in with the breath, reach the blood stream. This organ also contains the olfactory nerves, which transmit information about all smell to the brain, another important process by which essential oils interact with the body and mind.

The Urinary System

Essential oils can have a profound effect on the urinary system.

> Chamomile, Cedarwood and Juniper have an affinity with the kidneys, valuable for their tonic effect on these organs, and for use during kidney infections such as pyelitis and nephritis.
> The above oils, as well as Cypress, Eucalyptus, Fennel, Frankincense, Geranium and Rosemary, are useful diuretic oils, helpful where there is fluid retention or when the body needs to get rid of a lot of toxic waste.
> These oils should be used with care, however, and never for a long period, as they can mask serious conditions of the kidneys as well as disturbing the mechanisms that control fluid and salt balance through their effect of artificially increasing the amount of urine produced.
> Due to the fact that all the blood in the body passes through the kidneys twice in each hour, and the essential oils circulate in the body stream, great care should be taken with the amount of oils used, and the proper proportions should be adhered to, as excessive amounts can overload the kidneys causing them damage.
> A number of essential oils act as urinary tract antiseptics, the most valuable being Bergamot, Chamomile, Eucalyptus, Juniper, Sandalwood and Tea Tree, which can be applied in repeated hot compresses over the lower abdomen and can prove particularly helpful in treating cystitis.
> Camphor oil is described as being a good diuretic, and Thyme oil is also said to be effective against urinary tract infection.
> A number of essences, especially Chamomile and Geranium, are capable of effectively dissolving urinary stones.

The Reproductive System

Many oils can influence the reproductive system, both through their effects on the nervous system, and by stimulating the various glands involved in reproduction. Sterility, menstrual and menopausal problems, labor, frigidity, impotency, infections, and many other problems related to this system can be relieved using appropriate oils.

- Rose, Chamomile, Clary Sage, Cypress, Fennel, Jasmine, Lavender and Geranium are among those which have the most marked effects on this system, and can be used in a number of imbalances which arise due to physical or psychological disorder.
- Certain oils are reputed to have an aphrodisiac effect, particularly Jasmine and Ylang Ylang, and can be of particular help where problems arise due to emotional difficulties.
- Rose oil has a particular affinity with the female reproductive system, toning and cleansing the uterus, and regulating the menstrual cycle.
- Geranium has a balancing effect on hormonal secretion generally, and can also help to balance any irregularities in this regard.
- Rose oil is also reputed to increase the sperm count in men, and can be of value in cases of sterility due to this problem.
- Cases of frigidity and impotency are most often related to emotional factors, and oils which help to relieve stress and tension can be of particular help here, especially those which have the most exquisite scents, exerting a strong influence on the mind and emotions. Bergamot, Clary Sage, Neroli and Rose being particularly useful in this regard, as well as those mentioned previously.
- Menstrual cramps can be greatly relieved using certain antispasmodic oils, particularly Marjoram, Lavender and Chamomile.
- Many oils also have an emmenagogic effect and can help to bring on a period or increase scanty menstruation. These particular oils should never be used during pregnancy or where menstruation is normal or particularly heavy; Clary Sage, Myrrh, Sage, Basil, Juniper, Fennel and Rosemary being the most noted in this regard.
- Cypress, Geranium and Rose, due to their regulating effect, can help where periods are abnormally heavy, and Rosemary and Geranium can help reduce fluid retention which is often experienced some days before a period.
- Many of the essential oils which help with menstrual irregularities earlier in life can also be used to help minimize the physical and emotional problems associated with the menopause, particularly those which have a balancing and regulating effect on the hormones, such as Geranium and Rose.
- Chamomile and other antidepressant oils can help soothe and calm during menopause.

➤ Bergamot and Sandalwood can be effectively used to treat various infections associated with this system, and Bergamot in particular was found to be an excellent oil in preventing the spread of certain infections, including gonorrhea.

➤ Certain oils, particularly Jasmine, can induce labor by stimulating uterine contraction, helping to give a swift and relatively painless birth, although it should not be used during the actual months of pregnancy in case of miscarriage.

For problems related to the reproductive system, oils can be used in massage, hip baths, vaginal douches, or applied as compresses. They can also be used in aromatic burners, where problems may be due to emotional factors.

The Skin

The skin is the body's largest organ, covering nearly two square meters for the average adult. It is an organ of elimination and helps to purify the system by getting rid of wastes, which are carried in sweat through the pores of the skin. Sometimes when the kidneys or colon are not working as efficiently as they should, disorders of the skin can occur due to the excess toxins, which must then try and find an alternative route of elimination. The skin also acts as a barrier, protecting our internal organs and guarding against invading bacteria, and acts as a trigger to our senses between us and the environment. Another important function of the skin is the regulation of body temperature, cooling the body down by evaporation of sweat from its surface, or conserving heat when necessary.

Structurally, the skin is divided into 3 distinct layers;

♦ Epidermis – top layer
♦ Dermis – middle layer
♦ Subcutaneous – bottom layer

The top layer is called the epidermis and is made up of sheets of flattened cells which are either dead or dying, after being pushed up through the lower layers of the skin. These dead cells form keratin, a tough protein substance which is found in the hair and nails. Also present in the epidermis are cells which produce melanin, the pigment responsible for skin color.

The middle layer or the dermis consists of connective tissue which contributes to the support and elasticity of the skin. The dermis is much thicker than the epidermis, and also contains hair follicles, sebaceous glands, sweat glands, nerve endings, and blood vessels.

The innermost layer, the hypodermis or subcutaneous layer, serves as the receptacle for the formation and storage of fat, also acting as a support for blood vessels and nerves which pass to the more superficial parts of the skin. The hypodermis also contains bundles of involuntary muscle fibers which are attached to hair follicles and contract in response to fear or cold, thus causing the hair to stand erect.

The skin is vitally important in aromatherapy, because it is one of the two routes by which essential oils can get into the blood stream and thus travel around the body. How well the oils actually penetrate the skin and reach the blood stream can vary with each individual. Absorption will be delayed if the skin is blocked by toxins, either from the outside or inside. Fluid retention, cellulite and a lot of fatty tissue will also influence absorption rate.

The skin itself can benefit greatly from the use of essential oils. Appropriate oils can help to relieve many skin disorders, ranging from conditions such as dry, oily or dehydrated skins, to more serious disorders such as eczema, psoriasis and dermatitis. Massage alone, by stimulating blood flow and encouraging the delivery of fresh nutrients and oxygen, results in healthy cell growth, giving the skin a better texture and more radiant appearance. It helps to improve the skin's overall condition, tone and quality, and when combined with the use of essential oils, the results can be absolutely fantastic.

4
Aromatherapy for Babies & Children

Babies

 Aromatherapy can be used to advantage from the moment of birth, provided that a number of common sense precautions are borne in mind. It is vitally important that essential oils always be diluted before adding to the bath, as babies so often suck their thumbs or hands, and rub their fists into their eyes.

Undiluted essential oil forms a film on the surface of the water and can be very easily transferred via the hands to the face, mouth or eyes. Before adding to the bath, essential oils should be diluted in a few teaspoons of almond, soya or other bland oil, or up to a cup of milk (not skimmed), and mixed well. A single drop of Chamomile or Lavender will be sufficient in a baby bath to ease minor discomforts and aid sleep, once properly diluted. Regular addition of oils to the bath is a good preventative measure against nappy rash, preventing bacteria from developing on the skin for some time. Creams containing Calendula or Chamomile are very healing and helpful if nappy rash does become a problem. Calendula is particularly good if the skin is cracked and slow to heal.

To help with respiratory ailments, a drop of an appropriate oil may be placed on the sheet in the cot, or on their pajamas, so the baby will continually inhale the vaporized oil. Also, an essential oil could be sprayed or vaporized in the baby's room, to help ease coughs and congestion as well as encourage the baby to sleep. If placing a burner in the room, it should not be put too near the cot, but positioned a reasonable distance away, thus preventing the effects of the vapor from becoming too over powering, as well as ensuring that no accidents arise due to the burner being accidentally over turned.

Teething problems and the discomfort, and other health upsets associated with it, can be greatly minimized by the sensible use of essential oils. Chamomile is particularly useful at this time, with Lavender coming a close second. It is vitally important not to confuse Roman Chamomile with Moroccan Chamomile or German Chamomile. Moroccan Chamomile belongs to a different plant family altogether, and German Chamomile contains a much higher concentration of azulene, which only needs to be used in very small quantities. Neither of the latter oils is recommended for use on babies or children, and it is always advised that you alternate the use of Roman

Chamomile with Lavender oil, thus preventing possible residue build up in the babies system. Also, the body will cease to respond to a certain oil if it is used on a continuous basis. Other essential oil treatments should not be used continually, always allowing the baby or young child a reasonable break from the oils.

If teething problems should arise, diluted Chamomile oil, previously warmed, can be gently massaged onto the affected side of the face, extending the massage to include the area all around the ear. Sleeplessness caused by the discomfort can be aided by adding a drop of diluted Lavender oil to the bath, or by putting a drop of Lavender on the cot sheet or pajamas. Avoid using the same oil that was used in the facial massage.

Colicky pain can be reduced and the baby comforted by gently massaging the tummy or lower back in a clockwise direction, using diluted Chamomile or Lavender. It is of vital importance that no essential oils (even when they are diluted) be placed into a baby's mouth or ear. The same goes for children of all ages.

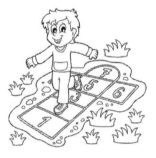

Children

Children generally respond very well to aromatherapy, as well as other natural forms of healing. This is partly due to the fact that they have no preformed expectations or prejudices about what is involved, and partly because their young bodies have excellent powers of recuperation, their powers of self healing not yet having been impaired by years of faulty diet, stress, unhealthy lifestyle, and environmental pollution, etc.

Certain safety precautions, however, must always be adhered to when using essential oils with children. An undiluted essential oil should never be used on a child, with the sole exception of very small amounts of Lavender on minor burns or injuries. Weaker dilutions of a blend should be prepared when mixing oil for massage, between 1% and 2% dilution, as opposed to a possible 3% dilution used for an adult.

When preparing a bath for a child, no more than 3 drops of an essential oil should be added, and always dilute the essence in a suitable carrier oil first. Inhalations should be given for only a few seconds initially, maybe half a minute to begin with, before increasing the time to a minute or two if the shorter inhalations are well tolerated. A young child should never be left alone with a bowl of hot water when receiving this treatment, but should be supervised the entire time. Essential oils should of course never be given by mouth, and all oils described as toxic or slightly toxic should be avoided.

The smaller body weight of a child enables the essential oils to bring about a beneficial effect more quickly than that of an adult, children also requiring much smaller doses. Coupled with the fact that their bodies have not yet been clogged by toxic accumulation that has built up over many years, the above factor makes for the use of essential oils in baths, inhalations, compresses, air sprays and massage. Colds, infections, illnesses, bruises, cuts, burns, grazes and insect bites, all causing pain and discomfort, can be effectively treated using essential oils.

The oils which are particularly suitable for use with children are Chamomile, Lavender, Rose, Benzoin, Mandarin, and also Peppermint in very small amounts. Eucalyptus and Tea Tree can be used in a burner, where any viral infection is present, and fevers can be relieved by gently sponging the child with 2 drops of Bergamot, or 2 drops of Chamomile added to a pint of water. This latter treatment can be used on a child aged 4 years and up.

You should never attempt to treat serious illnesses without referring to a medically qualified practitioner, and the doctor should be called immediately if the child is running a high temperature, is badly burnt, has convulsions or where there is any other sign that the child is in serious difficulty. If treating a minor condition which subsequently shows no sign of improving within 24 hours, a doctor or other medically qualified practitioner should be notified. Always observe the child for any physical or emotional changes while they are receiving essential oil treatment, especially after you have introduced a new oil in any form. A child is as individual as an adult, and even though an oil may be recommended as safe, there is a possibility that it may produce an allergic reaction, so always watch out for this. Always alternate the oils used, and do not treat the child with essential oils on a consistent basis, even though you may vary them. Be constantly alert when using essential oils in the presence of children and always follow certain safety precautions as regards placing the oil safely out of their reach after use, ensuring that the cap is securely tightened.

5
Essential Oils Description

❧ Angelica (Root) ❧

Strengthens the mind and spirit, helpful for those who are afraid, timid, and weak or who lack perseverance and have a tough time making decisions. Also strengthens physically, good for use in convalescence, particularly where conditions have been long, strength-depleting or chronic. Good for use after an operation or childbirth. A well known carminative, it can be used for flatulence, dyspepsia, also for a weak stomach and digestive system generally. Stimulates digestion, used for nausea, gastritis, hiccups, and stomach ulcers. Calms and balances nervous system. Good for poor blood circulations, particularly involving the lower extremities. Supports the formation of healthy blood cells, good for a weak heart. Used for colds, flu, sinus infections and chronic respiratory problems, for nose polyps intestinal infections. Supports immune system.

Properties:	Antiseptic, mild expectorant, stomach tonic, immuno-stimulant, carminative, blood circulation stimulant, adrenal gland sedative, strengthens mind and body, rejuvenates, anti-viral.
Blends with:	Bergamot, Clary Sage, Lemongrass, Juniper, Tea Tree.
Contraindications:	Not to be used before exposure to sunshine, sunbeds or ultra violet light.

❧ Basil (Herb) ❧

Clears the head, uplifts and stimulates, good for intellectual fatigue, aids concentration. Used for treating disorders of the respiratory and digestive systems, asthma, bronchitis, catarrh, hiccups, indigestion, vomiting, intestinal infections, gastroenteritis. Its value in these latter regards is more powerful if these conditions are of an emotional origin. Tones the nervous system both physically and emotionally, good for hysterics, indecision, depression, anxiety and nervous debility, also sciatica, neuritis, neuralgia and general nerve pains. A good oil for use in herpes, once not of the genitals, and can be used neat in the pre-blister stage. Stimulates and tones the skin, good for sluggish or congested skin, as an insect repellant, soothes wasp stings. Also good for tired, tight, overworked muscles and muscle spasm generally. Used for colds, earache, sinus, migraine, insomnia and balances secretions of the adrenal cortex.

Properties: Cephalic, antispasmodic, uplifting and stimulating, nerve tonic, antiseptic, expectorant, sudorific, emmenagogic.

Blends with: Lavender, Bergamot, Geranium, Petitgrain, Coriander.

Contraindications: Do not use during pregnancy or for anyone with sensitive skins.

❧ Benzoin (Benzoe Tree) ❧

Soothes irritated nerves, good for irritability, depression, stress, PMS, also warming and soothing, useful where there is sadness, loneliness or anxiety. Excellent for use in perfumes as a fixative, extends the shelf life of cosmetic preparations. Recommended for use as an inhalant for throat infections, coughs, bronchitis, colds, flu and sore throats, also loss of voice. Good for griping pains in the stomach and for urinary tract infections due to its ability to clear mucus, expel gas and stimulate the circulation. Extremely healing for many kinds of skin lesions, from cracked and chapped hands to chilblains. Wounds heal faster and hardened scar tissue softens with repeated application. Good for dry, rough and irritated skin, cleanses and protects the skin elasticity.

Properties: Soothing, stimulating, warming, comforting, balancing, calming, a natural fixative, antiseptic, expectorant, anti-inflammatory, diuretic, sedative.

Blends with: Rose, Geranium.

Contraindications: None, once used as recommended.

❧ Bergamot (Tree) ❧

Valuable for balancing the nervous system, used for tension, anxiety, depression, mood swings, refreshes and uplifts. Has an affinity with the urino-genital tract, used in cases of cystitis, urethritis, good where there is infection generally, the urinary tract, genitalia, mouth, skin, respiratory tract. Used for bronchitis, sore throats, tonsillitis, cold sores, herpes, ulcers, wounds, acne. Has a cooling effect during fevers, useful in cases of psoriasis and eczema, balances sebum production in oily or dry skin. Used to ease pain and discomfort of shingles and chickenpox. Helps relieve colic, flatulence, gastroenteritis, indigestion, balances appetite and may be helpful for sufferers of anorexia nervosa, or compulsive eaters. Excellent body deodorant, good for bad breath, good as a room fragrancer, an insect repellent. Small doses help to minimize many of the symptoms and side effects involved in uterine cancer. Widely used in the perfume industry.

Properties:	Nerve tonic, uplifting, balancing, antiseptic, febrifuge, deodorant, bactericide, anti-inflammatory, antidepressant, analgesic, antispasmodic, carminative, regulating, antiviral.
Blends with:	Lavender, Geranium, Ylang Ylang, Chamomile, Almost any flower oil.
Contraindications:	May cause skin irritation, not for use on extremely sensitive skins. Do not use before exposure to ultra violet light or rays.

❧ Black Pepper (Spice) ❧

A very warming oil used for muscular pain, stiffness and fatigue. Good for use before training or performance, for athletes and dancers, helps to prevent pain and stiffness and possibly improves performance. Used for marathon runners may improve time, and results in far less muscular fatigue. Also helps rheumatic and arthritic pain. Can be valuable in anemia, stimulates the spleen which is involved in the production of new blood cells. Can be of use following heavy bleeding or severe bruising. Stimulates the kidneys, but if used in too big an amount or for too long a period, it could cause damage to the kidneys. Particularly valuable for treating disorders of the digestive tract, used to treat a sluggish digestive system, also soothes the smooth muscle of the gut. If used in very small amounts it can help to bring down a high temperature.

Properties:	Warming, antispasmodic, carminative, tonic, stimulating, diuretic, rubefacient.
Blends with:	Rosemary, Lavender, Marjoram, Frankincense, Sandalwood.
Contraindications: can	Use in only small amounts and not over a long period of time, it may otherwise irritate the kidneys, causing damage. Use in low dilutions as it irritate the skin. Not for use on very sensitive skins.

❧ German Chamomile (Herb) ❧

Due to its much higher concentration of azulene, it may be preferred over Roman Chamomile for treatments of infections, wounds and skin disorders. Its anti-inflammatory powers make it of great value in treating colitis, gastritis and infections of the small intestine. It may be the better choice where wounds are particularly hard to heal, or where digestive disorders in adults are particularly chronic. However, due to the higher amount of azulene it contains, it cannot be recommended to be as safe for use as Roman Chamomile, which has an extremely low level of toxicity. German Chamomile, therefore, is not recommended for use with children, or where conditions are relatively mild, Roman Chamomile being a much better choice here, just as effective and without the toxic implications.

Properties: Medicinal properties overlap those of Roman Chamomile to a large extent.

Blends with: Rose, Lavender, Geranium, Bergamot, Petitgrain, Patchouli, Lemon.

Contraindications: Not for use with children due to the high amounts of azulene it contains, making is possibly toxic for them. Use in much smaller concentrations than those advised for its milder relative.

❧ Roman Chamomile (Herb) ❧

Used for anxiety, depression, insomnia, anger, irritability, fretfulness and other disorders linked with the mind and emotions. Good for any condition where inflammation is present, either internal or external. Good for disorders of the digestive system, flatulence, gastritis, indigestion, stomach ulcers, diarrhea, stimulates this system. Used for muscular aches and pains, arthritis and rheumatism, also helpful in menstrual disorders, painful periods, irregularity and the menopause. Good for earache, toothache, teething troubles and headaches. Used on the skin to help dermatitis, sensitive skins, wounds, dry skin, also acne. Stimulates the production of white blood cells, which help in our fight against disease. Good for use where there are allergies. The children's oil for hyperactivity, temper tantrums, aids sleep.

Properties: Soothing, calming, anti-inflammatory, antidepressant, nerve tonic, gastric tonic and stimulant, analgesic, leukocytosis, carminative, febrifuge, diuretic, hepatic, sedative, vasoconstrictor, vulnerary, sudorific.

Blends with: Rose, Lavender, Cedarwood, Melissa, Neroli, Geranium.

Contraindications: None, extremely low levels of toxicity making it suitable for use with children.

⊱ Cedarwood (Cedar Tree) ⊰

Used particularly for bronchial and urinary tract infections, cystitis, vaginal infections and discharges. Catarrhal conditions, especially chronic bronchitis. Used in skincare for its mildly astringent and antiseptic properties. Good for acne, also helpful for dandruff and other scalp problems, strengthening hair growth, good for oily hair, and hair loss. It helps calm during times of fear and nervous tension, reduces fear, aggression and anger, warms and comforts. For those who lack independence and for those who need courage. Has a tonic and stimulating action on the whole body, while at the same time reducing stress and tension. Traditional reputation as an aphrodisiac.

Properties: Antiseptic, mucolytic, astringent, aphrodisiac, expectorant, diuretic, calming, strengthening, rejuvenating, comforting, warming.

Blends with: Juniper, Neroli, Citrus Oils, Cypress, Petitgrain, Rose, Jasmine.

Contraindications: Not to be used during pregnancy in any form as it may have abortive effects.

⊱ Clary Sage ⊰

Has a relaxing effect, used for stress, tension, nervous anxiety, depression, a powerful muscular relaxant also, especially where muscular tension arises due to mental or emotional stress. Useful for treating asthma, also relieving anxiety which may cause or result from this disorder. Treats disorders of digestive system, cramps, colicky pains, flatulence. Also menstrual cramps, helps regulate scanty or missing periods. Good for female reproductive system generally, good for emotional problems in this regard too. A powerful tonic, useful in convalescence, after flu, depression, also post-natal. Prevents excessive sweating and reduces excessive production of sebum, especially on the scalp. Used for greasy hair, dandruff. Helps lower high blood pressure. Good for throat infections, coughs, asthma. Tones kidneys and stomach. Treats inflamed, mature, oily, dehydrated and normal skins. Useful for frigidity and impotency. Of particular value in stress related illnesses.

Properties:	Balancing, inspiring, revitalizing, relaxing, antidepressant, rejuvenating, aphrodisiac, uterine tonic, cuphoric, antispasmodic, warming, tonic, hypotensive, antiseptic, decongestive, anti-inflammatory, astringent, uplifting.
Blends with:	Cypress, Citrus Oils, Jasmine, Neroli, Juniper, Petitgrain, Geranium, Sandalwood.
Contraindications:	Not for use in pregnancy. Do not use before or after drinking alcohol. Be careful if driving as the oil can increase the effects of drunkenness.

❧ Cajeput (Tree) ❧

Useful for treating bronchial tract disturbances, especially colds, flu and bronchitis, when used in inhalations. Reduces the discomfort of sore throats and headaches that accompany colds. Dulls the pain of toothache. Beneficial for treating urinary tract infections, also helps remedy intestinal disorders, diarrhea, stomach cramps, nervous vomiting, and inflammations of the small intestine. Also benefits sufferers of rheumatism, neuralgia and earache. Can be used on compresses or as a chest rub. Always use well diluted as it can irritate the skin and never use alone in an inhalant before bedtime as it is a powerful stimulant. Supports the immune system.

Properties:	Analgesic, powerful stimulant, anti-inflammatory, antiseptic, bactericidal, mucolyptic.
Blends with:	Eucalyptus, Juniper.
Contraindications:	As it may irritate the skin it should not be used on people with very sensitive skin. Always use well diluted.

❧ Coriander ❧

Stimulates and aids digestion. May be helpful in treating anorexia nervosa. Relieves stomach and abdominal cramps, flatulence and hiccups. Good for neuralgia and rheumatic pains. A gentle stimulant when someone is tired and has low energy. Beneficial during convalescence and after a difficult childbirth. Also stimulates creativity and memory. Relaxes in a pleasant way during times of stress, irritability and nervousness. It may be beneficial for shock or fear. Helpful for scant, absent or painful menstruation.

Properties:	Digestive, stimulant, carminative, relaxant, emmenagogue, uplifting, calming, antispasmodic, analgesic, warming, comforting.
Blends with:	Rose, Jasmine, Sandalwood, Geranium, Citrus Oils.
Contraindications:	Do not use during pregnancy.

❧ Cypress (Tree) ❧

Useful for conditions involving an excess of fluid, incontinence, excessive perspiration, bleeding gums, bilious attacks and very heavy menstruation. Beneficial for use in skincare, treats oily or over hydrated skins, also acne, oily hair and dandruff. Treats piles/hemorrhoids, also varicose veins and chilblains. Softens the walls of hardened arteries and strengthens connective tissue. Tones the circulation, good where there is sluggishness in this regard. Sedates nerve endings of the respiratory system, use for asthma, whooping cough and emphysema. Regulates menstrual cycle, good for ovary problems, helps relieve painful periods, and reduces abnormally heavy loss. Useful in the latter regard in the early stages of the menopause. Balances female hormone system, helps reduce hot flashes of menopause. Use for diarrhea, excessive sweaty feet, nosebleeds, hemorrhage. Has a soothing effect on the nervous system in general, restoring calm, use for uncontrollable crying spells. For a weak bladder, also swollen feet. Internal and external bleeding. For those who avoid reality and become easily distracted.

Properties:	Astringent, antiseptic, antispasmodic, deodorant, expectorant, vasoconstrictor.
Blends with:	Juniper, Bergamot, Sandalwood, Clary Sage, Lavender, Citrus Oils.
Contraindications:	Not for use during pregnancy.

❧ Eucalyptus (Tree) ❧

Better known for its action on the upper respiratory tract, used for sinus problems, throat infections, colds, catarrh, influenza. Valuable for use during times of epidemic regarding disorders of this system. Use in inhalants or as a chest rub. Has a cooling effect on the body, used to reduce body temperature during fever. Its rubefacient action makes it of benefit in treating muscular aches and pains, also rheumatoid arthritis. Good for external wounds, particularly those that heal slowly, cold sores, the blisters in shingles, ulcers. Useful for most disorders of the urinary tract, including cystitis. Use for fluid retention especially where there is possible infection of toxemia. Treats facial neuralgia. Increases oxygen supply to everybody cell through its ability to activate red blood cell functioning thereby increasing oxygen bonding in the lungs, which is then passed to the rest of the body. Lowers blood sugar levels. A useful oil for treating diabetics due to the two latter properties.

Properties: Decongestant, expectorant, antiseptic, bactericidal, antiviral, febrifuge, rubefacient, diuretic, deodorant, stimulant, analgesic.

Blends with: Lemon, Lavender, Pine, Cypress, Melissa.

Contraindications: Do not use if receiving homeopathic treatment, may nullify the preparation. May cause skin irritation so only use in low dilutions.

❧ Fennel (Sweet) ❧

Relieves nausea, flatulence, indigestion, colic, hiccups, constipation, also decreases appetite, helpful for obesity. Water retention and accumulation of toxic wastes generally. Useful for treating cellulitis, gout and other inflammatory conditions of the joints, also helps treat alcoholism. Urinary tract antiseptic, used for retention of urine infections, may also help prevent kidney stones. Contains plant estrogens and has a marked effect on the female reproductive system, helps regulate the menstrual cycle, particularly where periods are scanty and painful, with cramping pains. Reduces symptoms of premenstrual stress and water retention associated with it. Stimulates production of estrogen by adrenal glands after ovaries have stopped functioning, reduces unpleasant symptoms of menopause. Estrogen helps maintain muscle tone, elasticity of skin and connective tissue, a healthy circulation and strong bones, so maintaining supply can postpone degenerative effects of aging. Can be taken as a tea. Add to face creams to improve skin condition. Also good for gum infections, increasing flow of breast milk, and eases coughs and colds.

Properties: Antispasmodic, anti-toxic, carminative, diuretic, antiseptic, expectorant, nerve tonic, tonic for digestive system.

Blends with: Lemon, Lavender, Geranium Sandalwood.

Contraindications: Not for use in epilepsy. Not for use with young children.

❧ Frankincense (Tree) ❧

Slows and deepens the breath, good for shortness of breath. Effects the mucus membranes, has a particular affinity for the pulmonary and genito-urinary tracts. Good remedy in all catarrhal conditions, used to treat coughs, bronchitis, asthma, laryngitis, also leucorrhea, gonorrhea, cystitis and nephritis. Useful for treating stomach and intestines generally. Use for hemorrhages, especially utering or pulmonary. A uterine tonic helpful for abnormally heavy periods. Safe to use during pregnancy. Use in skin care to help prevent wrinkles, helping to preserve a youthful complexion. Tones the skin, good to slack looking skin. Helps heal wounds, ulcers and reduce inflammation. Calms the emotions, breaks links with the past, helpful for people who dwell too much on past events, possibly leading to physical illness. Use for anxiety, tension, fear, obsession. Soothes and uplifts the mind.

Properties: Antiseptic, mucolytic, uterine tonic, astringent, anti-inflammatory, expectorant, calming, soothing, uplifting.

Blends with: Lavender, Myrrh, Neroli, Rose, Sandalwood, Citrus Oils.

Contraindications: None, once used as prescribed.

❧ Geranium ❧

Generally known for its balancing or normalizing effects on mind and body, which is due to its normalizing and regulating influence on the adrenal cortex. Useful for menopause and menstrual imbalance. Helps to balance the nervous system, use for anxiety, depression, and mood swings. Has a close relationship with the circulatory system helping to make blood more fluid. Dissolves hematosis due to its anti-coagulant properties. Stimulates circulation generally, enlarges capillaries, useful in cases of chilblains and mild frost bite. Useful in skincare, balances sebum production, use for dry or oily skin. Stimulates lymphatic system, good for lymphatic congestion generally, fluid retention, edema, and obesity. An aid to elimination, generally has a tonic effect on both the liver and kidneys, use to treat kidney stones, urinary tract infections and jaundice. Useful for treating wounds, ulcers, neuralgia, and various injuries. Indicated where there is an imbalance in hormone secretion. Uplifts and relaxes. A valuable insect repellant.

Properties: Calming, balancing, antidepressant, uplifting, antiseptic, astringent, diuretic, analgesic, sedative, hepatic, hemostatic.

Blends with: Most essences, especially Citrus Oils, Neroli, Juniper, Petitgrain, Lavender.

Contraindications: None, once used as prescribed.

❧ Ginger (Spice) ❧

Regulates moisture and raises body temperature, used for illnesses thought to be caused by cold and dampness, flu, rheumatism, colds, headaches, and muscle tension. Also diarrhea, catarrh and other conditions where the moisture originates within the body. Good for reducing motion sickness. Helps to prevent infectious illnesses, relieves stomach cramps, whether of digestive or menstrual origin and eases flatulence. Good for treating arthritis, rheumatism, general muscle pain and fatigue. High concentrations will irritate the skin, use in a low dilution. May be used as an aphrodisiac, said to treat male impotency.

Properties: Rubefacient, carminative, antispasmodic, aphrodisiac, antiseptic, warming, strengthening.

Blend with: Citrus Oils, Coriander, Patchouli.

Contraindications: None, once used as prescribed.

❧ Grapefruit (Tree) ❧

Particularly valuable for psychological conditions. Stimulates neuro-transmitters that cause a slight feeling of euphoria. Good where there is depression, lethargy, self doubt, confusion, frustration, envy or jealousy. Good for people who worry about the past, and who cannot let go. Also helps regulate eating disorders, both overeating and anorexia, particularly when due to psychological factors. Stimulates the liver and gall bladder. A beneficial treatment for oily skin and hair. Can be used in a blend for treating cellulite, giving a refreshing massage as well as increasing circulation and tightening the skin.

Properties: Hepatic, astringent, circulation stimulant, refreshing, uplifting, antidepressant.

Blends with: Clary Sage, Bergamot, Neroli, Lemon, Lavender, Geranium.

Contraindications: Do not use before sun exposure or exposure to any form of ultra violet light or rays.

❧ Hyssop (Herb) ❧

Good for chest infections where there is thick mucus. Helps to fluidify the catarrh so that it can be expelled more easily, good for coughs, bronchitis, calms persistent coughs. Use as a gargle for sore throats and loss of voice. Helpful in a cold compress for bruises, and a hot compress for rheumatism. Clears the mind, increases concentration, and stimulates creativity. Uplifts and provides direction. Due to its warming properties it can help to calm strong feelings and increase awareness. Said to bring inspiration and wisdom. Warms the stomach and helps stimulate digestion. Tones and strengthens the heart. Helpful with scanty or missing periods.

Properties:	Expectorant, cephalic, emmenagogue, uplifting, rejuvenating, warming.
Blends with:	Lavender, Sage, Rosemary, Clary Sage.
Contraindications:	Due to its cetone content it is a borderline oil in terms of toxicity, and should not be used by those with epileptic tendencies as it may trigger an attack. Do not use for people with high blood pressure and avoid during pregnancy. Best to choose a safer oil, although highly recommended for bruising.

❧ Jasmine (Climbing Bush) ❧

Works primarily on the emotional level and is of great value in psychological and psychosomatic problems. Use for depression, moodiness, apathy, listlessness, coldness, shyness and lack of confidence. Valued as an aphrodisiac, use for male impotency and rigidity. Has a marked effect on the female reproductive system, relieves uterine spasm, menstrual pain, relieves pain of childbirth and helps to promote the birth. Primarily of use for disorders of the nervous system and for use in conditions where aroma is important. Generally euphoric, has an uplifting effect while at the same time promoting calm and balance. Beautiful oil for skincare, use for dry, sensitive skins, redness or itching. Tones the skin, increases skin elasticity, helps prevent scarring and stretch marks. Can also be used for certain respiratory problems, catarrh, coughs, bronchial spasm, and breathing difficulties, particularly where these conditions have a 'nervous' origin.

Properties:	Aphrodisiac, antidepressant, sedative, euphoric, uplifting, uterine tonic, antiseptic, relaxing, warming.
Blends with:	Rose, Neroli, Sandalwood, Orange, Cypress.

Contraindications: Avoid during pregnancy as contraction of the uterus may result. Recommended for use during labour, however.

❧ Juniper (Tree) ❧

Has a special affinity to the urino-genital tract, having a purifying antiseptic and stimulant action on this system, use for cystitis, pyelitis, urinary stones, fluid retention, cellulitis. Dramatically relieves retention of urine, especially due to prostate enlargement, used in a small amount. Useful in cases of scanty, painful or missing periods. Use in the treatment of external hemorrhoids. Cleansing and detoxifying in many skin conditions, eczema, dermatitis, acne, psoriasis, particularly when there is 'weepiness', condition may worsen initially. Use in rheumatism, arthritis, gout, particularly where the condition is caused by, or aggravated by toxins in the tissues. Calms the nervous system, use for insomnia, fear, trembling, and anxiety. Mental cleansing, has an invigorating and clearing effect, use for lethargy, boredom or for someone who feels emotionally drained or confused after being in contact with a large number of people, or someone who was mentally draining.

Properties: Diuretic, emmenagogue, antiseptic, astringent, detoxifying, cleansing.

Blends with: Citrus Oils, Lavender, Cypress, Rosemary, Geranium.

Contraindications: Do not use during pregnancy.

❧ Lavender (Herb) ❧

Stimulates the lymphatic system, easing congestion and stimulating production of white blood cells. Combats effects of stress, use for anxiety, depression, general debility, irritability, palpitations. Regulates nervous system, inducing a relaxed state both physically and mentally. Good for aches and pains generally, rheumatism, sprains of the muscular system, headaches, earache, migraine. Stimulates regeneration of skin cells, use for burns, wounds, scar tissue, ulcers, acne, insect bites. Treats all catarrhal complaints, flu, nose and throat infections. Colic flatulence, indigestion. Use for sensitive skins, helps balance sebum production. Good for insomnia or any condition of emotional origin. Good for athlete's foot and ringworm. A useful insect repellant, relieves insect bites. Has a tonic and sedative action on the heart, helps reduce high blood pressure. Use for lymphatic congestion, cellulite, fluid retention, menstrual pain, pain of childbirth, strengthens contractions. A good all round oil. When in doubt, use Lavender. Heightens the action of other oils blended with it.

Properties:	Analgesic, antidepressant, bactericidal, decongestant, calming, soothing, balancing, antispasmodic, diuretic, antibiotic, sedative, anti-inflammatory, fungicidal, normalizing.
Blends with:	Most essences, especially Chamomile, Ylang Ylang, Fennel, Juniper, Marjoram.
Contraindications:	None. Its low level of toxicity makes it an ideal oil for use with children.

❧ Lemon (Tree) ❧

Useful in the treatment of external wounds and infections, illnesses due to its ability to stimulate the white blood corpuscles that defend the body against infection, use for bronchitis, flu, gastric infections, cuts, wounds, insect bites, boils. Helps to stop bleeding, good for minor injuries, after tooth extraction and for nose bleeds. A valuable mouthwash for toning gums, mouth ulcers and gingivitis. Helps maintain alkalinity in the system, good for gastric acidity, causing ulcers and pains, rheumatism, gout, and arthritis from acid buildup in the joints and soft tissue. Tones the digestive system, including the liver and pancreas. Tones the circulatory system, good for varicose veins, arteriosclerosis, high blood pressure, anemia and chilblains. Treats obesity due to congestion in the tissues. Use for colds, flu and catarrh. Brightens dull and discolored skin, may reduce freckles, acting as a mild bleach. Helps greasy skin, spots, broken capillaries, and wrinkles. Good for herpes, apply neat to remove corns, warts and verrucas, but avoid healthy skin.

Properties:	Febrifuge, Leukocytosis, hemostatic, bactericide, counteracts acidity.
Blends with:	Frankincense, Chamomile, Ylang Ylang, Bergamot, Petitgrain, Neroli, Ginger.
Contraindications:	Do not use before exposure to ultra violet light or rays. Use in low dilutions, and not on sensitive skin. Dilute before adding to a bath.

❧ Lemongrass (Tropical Grass) ❧

Has a powerful tonic and stimulating effect on the whole organism. Good for treating infectious illnesses and fevers. Soothes headaches, dilute before applying to temples. Good for use in the bath, for tired feet, and excessive sweating. Useful for treating skin with open pores and acne. Revitalizes, penetrates easily making skin and muscles supple and healthy. Good for tired legs and venous conditions. Improves energy and builds up resistance to fatigue. Induces a revitalizing process and is invigorating both physically and emotionally, good for boredom and lethargy. A good insect repellant. Stimulates lymph drainage and helps reduce swollen tissues. Stimulates the left brain, aids logical thinking and concentration. Use for intestinal tract disease, also strengthens blood vessels and helps prevent varicose veins. A good skin tonic, tightens weak connective tissue.

Properties: Antiseptic, bactericide, refreshing, stimulating, diuretic, astringent, tonic, cleansing, febrifuge.

Blends with: Eucalyptus, Juniper, Lavender, Geranium, Lime.

Contraindications: Do not use on sensitive skins. Dilute before adding to the bath. Not for use before exposure to ultra violet light or rays.

❧ Marjoram (Herb) ❧

Has a warming action on both the mind and body. Sedates the nervous system, producing calm. Use for anxiety, general debility, insomnia, irritability, stress, anger, also loneliness, bereavement and grief. Beneficial for treating asthma, bronchitis, colds, catarrh, coughs. A warm bath helps to ease chills and headache that accompanies flu. A vasodilator, it can be used to treat high blood pressure and other heart conditions. Valuable for treating digestive disorders, constipation, intestinal cramps due to its antispasmodic action, also menstrual cramps. Dilates the tiny capillaries just beneath the skin, producing a feeling of warmth, easing pain, and speeding healing in muscular problems, also reducing stiffness. Use for tired, tight, painful muscles, especially after physical exertion, also painful stiff joints, rheumatism, arthritis, general muscular pain, spasm, sprains, strain, also bruises and neuralgia. Warming on the emotional level, it can be used where there is loneliness and/or grief. As it lessens both physical and emotional response and sensation, it can calm excessive sexual drives. Good for migraine. Stimulates the parasympathetic nervous system.

Properties: Warming, comforting, analgesic, sedative, anti-aphrodisiac, rubefacient.

Blends with: Lavender, Bergamot, Rosemary, Rosewood.

Contraindications: Do not use during pregnancy. May be stupefying in large doses, so it should not be abused.

❧ Melissa (Lemon Balm) ❧

Sedates and uplifts, use for hysteria, tension, shock, over sensitivity, panic, anxiety, distress. Tones the heart, slows the heart, use for palpitations, high blood pressure, also calms over rapid breathing. Use for indigestion, flatulence, diarrhea, stomach pain, travel sickness, vomiting, and nausea. Has an affinity to the female reproductive system, a mild emmenagogue action, calms and regulates menstrual cycle, good for scanty and irregular periods, also sterility. Treats allergies, whether of the skin or respiratory system, use for eczema (low dilutions), asthma, and coughs. Cools in cases of fever, induces mild perspiration, of value in colds and influenza. Good for headaches, migraine, and temperature. Also bee and wasp stings. Generally regarded as a rejuvenating oil both physically and emotionally. Good for herpes, including genital. Stimulates the gall bladder and liver, regulates the digestive system. May benefit thyroid dysfunction.

Properties:	Antiviral, soothing, calming, antidepressant, uplifting, antispasmodic, febrifuge.
Blends with:	Rose, Neroli, Geranium, Lavender.
Contraindications:	Do not use during pregnancy. Do not use on sensitive skins. Otherwise always use in low dilutions.

❧ Mandarin (Tree) ❧

Good for treating digestive disorders, has a tonic and stimulant effect on the stomach and liver. Also for gall bladder problems, and has a calming effect on the intestines, use with other citrus oils for best results, gently massage into tummy in a clockwise direction. Use for pre menstrual syndrome, good for menstrual cramps as well as emotional problems related to it. Relaxes and uplifts, use for tension, fear, sadness, anxiety, irritability and insomnia. Good for use during convalescence, especially after an emotional illness, and an excellent oil for treating children. Use this gentle oil for childhood disorders, tummy upsets, hiccups, irritability. Good for any fragile individual, use for the elderly.

Properties:	Hepatic, calming, cheering, inspiring, strengthening, relaxing, stomach tonic, antispasmodic.
Blends with:	Lavender, Neroli, Sandalwood, Bergamot, Coriander, Citrus Oils.
Contraindications:	Not for use before exposure to ultra violet light or rays.

❧ Myrrh (Tree) ❧

Highly valued as a healer of wounds, especially those that are slow to heal. Use for weeping skin conditions such as eczema and athlete's foot. Heals cracked and chapped skin, good for use on cracked heels and hands. Heals gum disorders and mouth ulcers, very good for the gums generally. Treats chest infections, catarrh, chronic bronchitis, colds and sore throats. Dries excess mucus. Tonic and stimulating action on the stomach and the whole digestive tract, use for diarrhea, gentle clockwise massage. Use as a vaginal douche against thrush, eliminates itch and discharge. Use as an external application for hemorrhoids.

Properties: Antiseptic, healing, anti-inflammatory, expectorant, astringent, emmenagogue, antifungal.

Blends with: Frankincense, Sandalwood, Cedarwood, Patchouli, Coriander, Ginger.

Contraindications: Not to be used during pregnancy.

❧ Neroli (Orange Tree) ❧

Has a pronounced effect on the nervous system and is used for anxiety, stress, anger, irritability, shock, and palpitations. Primarily of use where problems are of an emotional origin. Also valuable for use in hysteria, insomnia due to anxiety, fear, hypertension and panic. Relieves spasm in smooth muscle particularly that of the intestines. Beneficial for flatulence and diarrhea due to nervous tension, also good for nervous disorders of the heart. Valuable for use in skin care, it stimulates the growth of healthy new cells having a rejuvenating effect, use for prematurely aging skin, dry, sensitive skins, broken capillaries and thread veins. Improves skin elasticity, also having a bactericidal effect on the skin. Reputed aphrodisiac - the quality of this oil stems from its ability to calm any nervous apprehension that may be experienced in this regard. Has an exquisite scent and is widely used in commercial perfumery. Good to prevent stretch marks.

Properties: Sedative, calming, antispasmodic, bactericidal, antiseptic, antidepressant, skin regenerative.

Blends with: Citrus Oils, Chamomile, Rosewood, Lavender, Frankincense, Sandalwood, Cedarwood.

Contraindications: None, once used as prescribed.

❧ Niaouli (Tree) ❧

Good for all respiratory tract infections, treats colds, flu, bronchitis and coughs, and other nose, throat or chest infections. Use in chest rubs or inhalants, not late in the evening as it is a powerful stimulant. Also beneficial for treating infections of the urinary tract. Aids wound healing by stimulating tissue renewal, use for minor wounds, burns, cuts and grazes, particularly if any dirt has gotten into them at the time of injury. Good for the treatment of acne and boils. Niaouli is a cousin of Cajeput, but unlike the latter, it is not a skin irritant, and is well tolerated by the skin and mucus membranes when used in suitable dilutions. Has been used topically to treat rheumatic pain.

Properties: Antiseptic, tissue stimulant, stimulant, healing, analgesic.

Blends with: Lemon, Orange, Eucalyptus, Hyssop, Lavender.

Contraindications: None, once used as prescribed.

❧ Orange (Tree) ❧

Valuable for constipation as well as diarrhea, due to its normalizing effect on the peristaltic action of the intestines. Benefits the heart by lowering the heart rhythm, treats cardiac spasm. Calms, relaxes and regenerates the nervous system, use for tense, nervous, withdrawn people. Influences mood, positively and joyfully, harmonizes feelings and awakens creativity. Benefits and soothes dry, irritated or acne prone skins, use well diluted. Good for aging, rough or calloused skins, having a regenerative effect. Softens the epidermis and stimulates circulation, good for skin that lacks sufficient blood circulation or remains cold. Stimulates lymph fluids, use for cellulitis and swollen tissues, also fluid retention. Stimulates the digestive system including the gall bladder, also the kidneys and bladder. Helps to reduce fever. Use for gingivitis, a general gum tonic and mouth ulcers.

Properties: Antidepressant, antispasmodic, mild sedative, febrifuge, warming, balancing, stimulating, heart tonic, diuretic, cholagogue.

Blends with: Frankincense, Coriander, Ginger, Sandalwood, Cypress, Ylang Ylang.

Contraindications: Do not use before exposure to ultra violet rays or light. May irritate the skin, dilute before adding to a bath. Caution on people with sensitive skin.

❧ Patchouli (Herb) ❧

Good for use in skin care, treats acne, cracked skin, certain types of eczema, fungal infections such as athlete's foot, some skin allergies, and dandruff. Also beneficial in the healing of wounds and can be used to treat yeast infections of the mouth and vagina. Has been used to treat obesity, and to induce loss of appetite and reduce fluid retention. Repels insects, use to treat insect bites. Said to have aphrodisiac qualities but this will depend on the person's aroma preference, some people find the odor of Patchouli repugnant. Can be used for treating anxiety or depression, small quantities were found to have an uplifting effect, but larger doses tended to sedate. Dries weeping sores and wounds, regenerates skin cells in much the same way as Lavender and Neroli. Used in perfumes, acts as a natural fixative.

Properties:	Antiseptic, febrifuge, stimulant, tonic, anti-inflammatory, fungicidal, cell regenerator, antidepressant, insecticide, aphrodisiac.
Blends with:	Bergamot, Geranium, Lavender, Myrrh, Neroli, Rose, Ginger.
Contraindications:	None, once used as prescribed.

❧ Peppermint (Herb) ❧

Use as a remedy for digestive upsets, colic, diarrhea, indigestion, nausea, vomiting and stomach pain. Has a beneficial action on the stomach, liver, and intestines, relieves smooth muscle spasm in the stomach and gut. Use well diluted in a clockwise direction, massage on abdomen. Peppermint tea can also be helpful. Treats colds and influenza, has a cooling effect in feverish conditions, also inducing sweating – refreshing and cooling after a hot day. Good for treating sunburn. Cleanses and encourages toxic elimination of the skin, use for irritated skins, toxic congestions, inflammation, acne, as an insect repellant. Benefits sinusitis, bronchitis, catarrh, coughs, flu. Clears the head, use for mental fatigue, memory and concentration. Stimulates the nervous system, good for treating shock, also neuralgia and general debility. Will disturb sleep if used late in the evening.

Properties:	Antispasmodic, cephalic, warming, stimulating, febrifuge, antiseptic, analgesic, decongestant, insecticide.
Blends with:	Lavender, Rosemary.
Contraindications:	Do not use in conjunction with homeopathic remedies as it may nullify the effects of same. Do not use during pregnancy. May cause skin irritation.

❧ Petitgrain (Bitter Orange Tree) ❧

Similar to Neroli, but not as potent therapeutically. Produces a balancing effect on the mind and emotions, relaxes but at the same time uplifts and revitalizes. Produces a positive effect when people are feeling sad or disappointed. Useful for depression, less acute anxiety etc. Neroli should be used where emotional disorders are more severe, or the two oils could be blended together. Petitgrain is cleansing and revitalizing when used on the skin, as a bath oil or shower gel. In massage oils and facial lotions it tightens and cleanses the skin, use for acne or edema of the skin.

Properties: Stimulating, balancing, relaxing, calming, antidepressant, mildly sedating, refreshing, cleansing, revitalizing, uplifting.

Blends with: Rosemary, Lavender, Geranium, Bergamot.

Contraindications: Do not use before exposure to ultra violet light or rays.

❧ Rose ❧

Excellent for treating disorders of the female reproductive system, cleansing, purifying and regulating, has a tonic effect on the uterus, good where there is loss of uterine muscle tone. Regulates menstrual cycle, cleanses wounds of impurities, and reduces excessive loss. Said to increase semen production. Useful for mental and emotional problems relating to this. Use in cases of sterility for males and females, helps lift the mind, good for depression (also post natal), moodiness, lack of confidence, frigidity, male impotency, insomnia. Tones and promotes circulation, cleanses the blood, relieves cardiac congestion, tones capillaries, regulates the action of the spleen and heart. Tones the stomach, promotes flow of bile, use for liver problems, constipation, nausea, vomiting. Calms nervous system, use for tension, stress, fatigue, lethargy, peptic ulcers, and heart disease arising from stress. Use on dry, sensitive or aging skins, redness and inflammation, thread veins.

Properties: Uterine tonic, antidepressant, aphrodisiac, balancing, regulating, astringent, antiseptic, uplifting, tonic.

Blends with: Many essences, especially Sandalwood, Frankincense, Patchouli, Clary Sage.

Contraindications: None, said to be the least toxic of all essences. Use as prescribed.

❧ Rosemary (Herb) ❧

Has a marked effect on the nervous system, use where there is loss of function due to sensory or motor nerve impairment – loss of smell, poor sight, and speech impairment. An excellent brain stimulant, improves memory, clears the head generally, use in cases of mental fatigue or lethargy, confusion and doubt, aids concentration. Use for pain of headache, migraine, rheumatism. Tones the heart, especially where palpitations occur due to a nervous disorder. Helps to normalize blood pressure (low). Normalizes cholesterol levels in the blood, use for atherosclerosis. Good for lymphatic congestions, use where there is fluid retention once it is not due to a kidney problem. Also obesity and cellulitis, stimulates circulation generally. Use for arthritis, rheumatism, gout aches and pains generally. Stimulates digestion, also treats intestinal infection and diarrhea, use for colitis, flatulence, stomach pains, liver and gall bladder disorders, also respiratory disorders, asthma, catarrh, bronchitis, sinusitis. Cleanses congested skins, use on wounds. Has a special affinity to water, use for scalp disorders, dandruff and hair loss, as a rinse. Add to shampoo.

Properties:	Stimulant, analgesic, diuretic, antispasmodic, carminative, antiseptic, nerve tonic, strengthening.
Blends with:	Cedarwood, Frankincense, Herbal Oils.
Contraindications:	Do not use on people who suffer from high blood pressure, or for those susceptible to epileptic fits.

❧ Rosewood (Tree) ❧

Has a tonic effect on the body without being a stimulant, very good tonic for the autonomic nervous system, helps relieve tiredness, nervousness and stress. Mildly analgesic, it is effective in clearing headaches, especially if they are allied to slight nausea. Clears the head, steadies the nerves, useful during exams or when driving long distances. Calms, while at the same time, has an uplifting effect on the mind and emotions, useful at times of crisis, where a clear head and calm logical thinking is required. May have an aphrodisiac effect due to its influence on the mind and emotions. Good for use in the bath or as a massage oil. Mainly used in the manufacture of bath and skincare products. Particularly effective for treating dry skin.

Properties:	Antibacterial, deodorant, mildly analgesic, calming, uplifting, aphrodisiac, tonic.
Blends with:	Marjoram, Lavender, Bergamot, Lemon, Frankincense, Geranium.

Contraindications: None, once used as prescribed.

❧ Sage (Herb) ❧

Best known for its affinity to the muscular system, often referred to as the 'sports therapist's oil', use for fibrositis, torticollis, torn ligaments and tendons, over exercised muscles, suitable for all states of fatigue, particularly after strenuous effort. Dissolves uric acid crystals which build up in sport, softens muscles. Also good for rheumatoid arthritis, aches and pains generally. Useful in cases of obesity due to congestion and fluid retention. Treats ulcers, wounds, congested skin. Clears the senses and improves memory. A general stimulant said to be a good nerve tonic. Has a powerful action on the female reproductive system, induces menstruation, and promotes the birth of a baby during labor, inducing uterine spasm. Can clear headaches, use in very low dilutions in gargles and mouth washes for mouth and throat infections.

Properties: Diuretic, emmenagogue, nerve tonic, antispasmodic, stimulant, antiseptic, astringent.

Blends with: Lavender, Rosemary, Marjoram.

Contraindications: Do not use on anyone suffering from high blood pressure or on those susceptible to epileptic fits or convulsions. Do not use in pregnancy. Large amounts are toxic to the nervous system and may produce paralysis, also severe and violent uterine spasm. Clary Sage presents a much safer oil to use, offering much the same properties as Sage.

❧ Sandalwood (Tree) ❧

A most effective, sedative oil, has a very relaxing effect as well as being slightly uplifting, use for anxiety, tension, depression, insomnia, stress. Useful for treating genito-urinary infections and conditions, especially where there is mucus discharge or inflammation of the mucus membrane, cystitis, gonorrhea, urethritis. Also useful in these regards, in relation to respiratory disorders, dry persistent cough, sore throat, bronchitis, laryngitis, catarrh, hiccups. A valuable expectorant where congestion is present in this system. Also good where there is intestinal spasm and/or inflammation, colic, diarrhea, gastritis, nausea, vomiting. A valuable fixative in many high class perfumes, highly valued for its cosmetic properties. Beneficial to many skin types and skin problems, tends to balance production of sebum, use for dry and dehydrated skin, also acne and oily skin, treats thread veins. Long held reputation as an aphrodisiac, probably ties in with its use in the perfume industry.

Properties:	Sedative, relaxing, slightly uplifting, antiseptic, mild analgesic, antispasmodic, mucolytic, expectorant, aphrodisiac, warming, tissue regenerative, harmonizing.
Blends with:	Most essences, especially Rose, Ylang Ylang and Neroli.
Contraindications:	None, once used as prescribed.

❧ Tea Tree (Tree) ❧

A powerful immuno-stimulant, enhancing and potentiating the body's defenses. Good for infectious illnesses such as colds, flu, bronchitis, sore throat, and other infectious conditions of the respiratory tract. Use on the skin to treat cold sores, blisters of shingles and chickenpox, verruca, warts, acne, athlete's foot, ringworm, candida, infected wounds and insect bites. Can be used neat on cold sores in the pre blister stage, also shingles and chickenpox warts. Helps to control the candida organisms by reducing the rate at which they reproduce, and also by strengthening the body's ability to resist them. Good for thrush. Helps the digestive system by controlling candida albicans in the gut. Also good for gastritis and indigestion. Use in bath and massage for patients, some weeks prior to operations, will help build up their defense. Due to its powerful effect on the immune system it has been used in connection with the treatment of AIDS patients.

Properties:	Bactericidal, antiviral, fungicidal, immuno-stimulant, antiseptic, decongestant.
Blends with:	Lemon, Lavender.
Contraindications:	May irritate the skin and should therefore be used with caution on sensitive skins.

❧ Thyme (Herb) ❧

Useful for people with a sluggish digestive system or to strengthen the body during convalescence. Valuable for use with gastric infections, also expels intestinal worms. Treats colds, coughs and sore throats, use for mouth, nose, throat and chest infections. Useful for all infections of the urinary tract, also acting as a diuretic. Stimulates the production of white blood corpuscles so strengthening the body's resistance to invading organisms. Stimulates the circulation generally and raises low blood pressure, use for fatigue, depression and lethargy. Stimulates the brain and improves memory, as it can produce a balancing effect, it may also be of help with insomnia. Stimulates the appetite, useful after an illness. Good for sores and wounds, also insect bites and stings. Can be used to relieve rheumatic pain. Treats weak or missing periods, stimulates menstruation.

Properties:	Digestive stimulant, antiseptic, diuretic, leukocytosis, hypertensive, strengthening, antibacterial, antispasmodic, emmenagogue.
Blends with:	Bergamot, Lemon, Melissa and Rosemary.
Contraindications:	Do not use in pregnancy. Do not use on anyone suffering from high blood pressure. Not for use on sensitive skins. Always dilute well, even before adding to the bath. Not for use on people with epileptic conditions or hyperthyroidism.

❧ Ylang Ylang (Tree) ❧

A heart regulator, and can be used to slow an over rapid heartbeat (tachycardia). Helps to lower high blood pressure. Also capable of slowing over rapid breathing (hyperpnea), which may tie in with its sedative action on the autonomic nervous system. Use for anxiety, shock, fright or extreme anger, very calming after an emotional upset, which may have been the cause of the above physical symptoms. Comforting at times of bereavement. Its calming and relaxing effect may be responsible for its reputation as an aphrodisiac, use for impotency and frigidity, also inner coldness. Good for use on the abdomen for gastroenteritis and other digestive disorders including those which might arise due to a nervous or emotional upset. Very extractive and draws out impurities, treats oily and congested skins. Balances the secretion of sebum, and can also be of benefit to dry skins. Good for insomnia, nervous depression, low self confidence, tension headaches. Good for relaxing tense muscles due to stress.

Properties: Antiseptic, hypotensive, balancing, calming, aphrodisiac, sedative, antidepressant and relaxing.

Blends with: Most essences, especially Patchouli, Sandalwood, Bergamot and Lemon.

Contraindications: None. However if used in too high a concentration for too long a time, it can give rise to nausea and/or headache. Always use a prescribed.

6
Blending & Carrier Oils

Essential oils are too powerful and too highly concentrated to be used on their own, so they must be diluted in a carrier oil before being used in aromatherapy.

Carrier oils are classed as fixed oils because, unlike essential oils, they do not evaporate and therefore provide an excellent base for aromatherapy blends. They contain an array of vitamins, minerals, essential fatty acids and proteins, and have a wide range of benefits including;

♦ The treatment of dandruff
♦ Softening and smoothing the skin
♦ Tightening of the tissues
♦ Soothing inflamed skin
♦ Treating eczema and psoriasis
♦ Reducing scarring after operations
♦ Useful for treating wrinkles
♦ Useful for treating cellulite

The importance of choosing a carrier oil must not be underestimated. 98% of the blend will consist of the carrier oil so it vital to choose one that matches your particular needs at that time. Before you can choose, it is important to know some basic facts about the properties, viscosity, and advantages and disadvantages of each carrier oil so you feel completely confident in your choice.

Recommended carrier oils:

Sweet Almond Oil	*Jojoba Oil*
Apricot Kernel Oil	*Macadamia Oil*
Avocado Oil	*Olive Oil*
Borage Seed Oil	*Peanut Oil*
Coconut Oil	*Sesame Oil*
Evening Primrose Oil	*Soya Bean Oil*
Grapeseed Oil	*Sunflower Oil*
Hazelnut Oil	*Wheatgerm Oil*

❧ Sweet Almond Oil ❧

*not to be confused with Bitter Almond which is toxic

Color: Pale yellow
Viscosity: Medium – easily absorbed into the skin
Properties: Rich in vitamins (A, B1, B2, B6, D), minerals, linoleic, oleic, palmitic, linolenic and stearic acids.
Uses: Often regarded as the most widely used carrier oil, Sweet Almond is suitable for all skin types. It helps to soften and nourish the skin, helps to soothe inflammation or irritation and helps to revitalize skin.

❧ Apricot Kernel Oil ❧

Color: Pale yellow
Viscosity: Medium – rich but light and easily absorbed into the skin
Properties: High in vitamins (A, B1, B2, B6, B17, E) and linoleic, oleic and palmitic acids.
Uses: A rich, nourishing carrier oil suitable for all skin types. Helps to revitalize and moisturize the skin.

❧ Avocado Oil ❧

Color: Dark olive green
Viscosity: Thick – luxurious, rich texture absorbed into the upper layers of skin
Properties: Rich in vitamins (A, B1, B2, D, E), lecithin, minerals, protein and linoleic, oleic, palmitic and linolenic acids.
Uses: Containing healing and regenerative properties, Avocado Oil is ideal for dry skin conditions such as eczema and psoriasis. It softens and smoothes the skin and helps to reduce wrinkles.

❧ Borage Seed Oil ❧
*commonly known as starflower oil

Color:	Pale yellow
Viscosity:	Thin to medium
Properties:	Borage Seed Oil has the highest concentration of Gamma Linolenic Acid (GLA) naturally available in any plant source. It also contains vitamins (A, B1, B2, B6, D, E), oleic and linoleic acids.
Uses:	GLA, an Omega-6 essential fatty acid, combats inflammation, eczema, dermatitis, asthma, arthritis, diabetes and obesity. Borage Seed Oil is suitable for all skin types.

❧ Coconut Oil ❧

Color:	Clear
Viscosity:	Thin – easy to spread and non-oily
Properties:	A rich source of Omega 3, 6, 9 as well as vitamins (A, B1, B2, E) and minerals.
Uses:	Acts as an emollient to soothe and soften the skin, helps to relieve dry, itching skin, helps to prevent premature aging and is an excellent treatment for dry scalp.

❧ Evening Primrose Oil ❧

Color:	Pale yellow
Viscosity:	Thin
Properties:	Contains a high essential fatty acid content, consisting primarily of Omega-6 Gamma Linoleic Acid (GLA). Also a rich source of vitamins (B1, B2, B6, E) and minerals.
Uses:	Excellent in treating many skin conditions such as eczema, psoriasis, rosacea, flaky skin, dandruff, skin aging and inflammation. It is also useful for PMT.

❧ Grapeseed Oil ❧

Color:	Virtually clear with a slight green tinge
Viscosity:	Thin – light texture that is easily absorbed into the skin
Properties:	Rich in linoleic acid plus vitamins (A, B, E), antioxidants and minerals.
Uses:	Has slight astringent properties, therefore helping to tighten and tone the skin. It is suitable for all skin types and is widely used as a base for massage blends.

❧ Hazelnut Oil ❧

Color:	Yellow
Viscosity:	Thin – light texture that is easily absorbed by the skin
Properties:	A rich source of oleic acid along with smaller amounts of linoleic and palmitic acids, contains vitamins (A, B, D, E) and minerals.
Uses:	Contains astringent properties making it ideal for oily, acne skin, encourages cell regeneration and stimulates circulation.

❧ Jojoba Oil ❧

Color:	Golden yellow
Viscosity:	Medium – light, silky texture that deeply penetrates the skin
Properties:	Rich in vitamin E and also contains vitamins A, B1, B2 & B6.
Uses:	Chemically similar to that of the skin's own oil (sebum) making it ideal for use on oily or dry skin due to its balancing properties.

❧ Macadamia Oil ❧

Color:	Pale yellow
Viscosity:	Thick – easily absorbed by the skin
Properties:	High in palmioleic acid, also contains proteins, minerals and vitamins (A, B1, B2, B6, C, E).
Uses:	Excellent anti-aging properties, softens and heals the skin, great strengthening and nourishing treatment for the hair.

❧ Olive Oil ❧

Color: Olive Green

Viscosity: Thick – leaves an oily coating on the skin

Properties: Rich in antioxidants, vitamins, minerals, nutrients and oleic, palmitic, linoleic and linolenic acids.

Uses: The antioxidants help to neutralize free radicals, repairing skin damage and preventing skin aging. Olive oil is a fantastic emollient used for nourishing the skin and promoting wound healing.

❧ Peanut Oil ❧

Color: Pale yellow

Viscosity: Thick – leaves an oil coating on the skin

Properties: Rich in vitamin E, oleic and linoleic acids.

Uses: Suitable for all skin types, particularly dry skin.

❧ Sesame Oil ❧

Color: Pale yellow

Viscosity: Medium to thick – spreads easily

Properties: Rich in essential fatty acids such as linoleic, oleic, palmitic and linolenic acids, as well as protein, vitamins (A, B1, B2, B6, D) and minerals.

Uses: Suitable for all skin types, particularly dry skin, eczema and psoriasis. Contains a natural SPF so helps to protect the skin from harmful UV rays.

❧ Soya Bean Oil ❧

Color: Pale yellow

Viscosity: Thin to medium – light texture that is easily absorbed by the skin

Properties: Naturally rich in essential fatty acids, lecithin, sterolins and vitamin E, it also contains vitamins A & C.

Uses: Soya Bean Oil has excellent skin conditioning qualities and is useful as a treatment for inflamed and irritated skin. Suitable for all skin types.

❧ Sunflower Oil ❧

Color: Pale yellow
Viscosity: Thin – light texture that penetrates easily into the skin
Properties: High in vitamins A, D & E, linoleic acid, protein and minerals.
Uses: Suitable for all skin types and helps to relieve eczema and psoriasis.

❧ Wheatgerm Oil ❧

Color: Orange – brown
Viscosity: Thick – leaves a sticky residue on the skin
Properties: Very high vitamin E content, plus essential fatty acids such as linoleic and oleic acids.
Uses: Recommended for use on scarring and problem dry skin. Often used to prevent stretch marks. Due to its high vitamin E content it acts as a natural preservative in any homemade blends.

7
How to Use Essential Oils in the Home

The uses of essential oils in the home are endless and can be easily incorporated into everyday living in a variety of different ways. Whether you would like to enjoy a relaxing bath, create a beautifully scented, natural air freshener or lavish a rich moisturizing oil all over your body, essential oils offer the perfect opportunity to create your own perfect lotions and potions.

Some of the most popular ways to use essential oils include the following;

In the Bath

This is probably the easiest and most effective way to implement aromatherapy into your lifestyle, and is a perfect place for beginners to start. The relaxing warm water complements the oil and can provide relief from;

♦ Stress-related conditions
♦ Tension and anxiety
♦ Muscle pain and stiffness
♦ Restlessness

Remember, though, that essential oils do not dissolve in water and should therefore be mixed with a carrier oil or a small amount of unperfumed soap or shower gel. To use essential oils in the bath;

➢ Run a hot bath (but not too hot) and close all doors and windows (to contain the scent).
➢ Add appropriate drops of essential oil to 10mls of carrier oil.
➢ Add the blend to the water. Using your hand, swirl the water around to disperse the oils.
➢ Sit back, soak and relax.

Massage

With the wide array of therapeutic properties offered by essential oils, their popularity in massage comes as no surprise. Massage in its own right offers many fantastic benefits to both our body and mind, but when you throw essential oils into the mix, these benefits are dramatically enhanced.

Aromatherapy massage is effective in;

♦ Promoting a good night's sleep
♦ Reducing stress and tension in the body
♦ Improving circulation which in turn eliminates toxins from the body at a faster rate
♦ Reducing inflammation
♦ Soothing dry, itchy, irritated skin
♦ Helping to fight signs of aging

The essential oils should be blended with a carrier oil and while some dilutions will contain less or more essential oils, the following dilutions can be used as a guideline;

Treatment Area	No. of Drops of Essential Oil	Quantity of Carrier Oil
Skin Care (Face & Neck Massage)	4 – 10	15ml (1 tablespoon)
Specific Area, e.g. hand or elbow	4 - 10	15 ml (1 tablespoon)
Full Body Massage	10 – 20	30 ml (2 tablespoons)

Compress

A compress is a piece of material, typically a muslin cloth or a soft face cloth, that is soaked in either hot or cold water, and applied directly to a specific part of the body. A cold compress is traditionally used to treat localized swelling, joint sprains, headaches and insect bites. Meanwhile, a hot compress is more suitable for muscular aches and pains, earache, toothache and menstrual cramps.

To make a compress;

➢ Fill a bowl with 200 ml of hot or cold water.
➢ Add 5 - 8 drops of the chosen essential oil.

> Soak the muslin/face cloth in the bowl of water for approximately 60 seconds. Make sure the material is completely saturated.
> Remove the material, squeeze out any excess water and apply over the affected area.
> Hold the compress in place by using either your hand, or wrap a bandage or cling film around it.
> Leave in place for approximately 2 hours.
> Remove and repeat as often as is necessary.

Inhalation

Adding essential oils to a bowl of steaming water is a potent way to treat upper respiratory tract disorders such as colds, flu, sinusitis or blocked nose (not recommended for asthmatics). It is also an effective way to treat oily skin, helping to unclog pores, remove excess sebum from the skin and brighten the complexion. To make a stream inhalation;

> Fill a large bowl with boiling water.
> Add 4 - 8 drops of your chosen oil.
> Lean over the bowl with a towel covering your head in such a way that the sides are closed over (this helps to seal the aroma). Do not lean too close as you could burn yourself.
> Close your eyes and breathe through your nose for 4 – 5 minutes. Take deep, slow breaths.

Vaporizer

Vaporising/Diffuser using essential oils involves vaporizing the oils in a variety of devices into the surrounding air. The most popular device is a ceramic vaporizer or burner. At the top of the burner there is a small bowl (for water and the essential oils) and at the bottom there is an area where you place a small candle. The heat from the candle evaporates the water above, creating an aroma that dissipates around the room. Burners can be used to;

♦ Relax and calm
♦ Uplift
♦ Create mental clarity
♦ Strengthen focus and concentration
♦ Act as an insect repellent

Other popular methods of vaporizing include using a diffuser, a light bulb ring or a warm radiator (place 2 drops of essential oil on a cotton pad and place on the radiator).

8
Choosing Essential Oils

Choosing the finest pure essential oils is an extremely important factor in determining how effective the aromatherapy blend or treatment will be, and with the large selection of essential oils available on the market along with a growing number of suppliers, this task can be a daunting one. Before choosing an essential oil brand, it is important to carry out an adequate amount of research first, taking into account the following considerations;

♦ Purity
♦ Quality
♦ Price
♦ Storage

Purity
Choose oils that are 100% essential oils, ones that are not synthetics, dilutions or adulterations. Avoid terms such as "nature-identical", "fragrance oil" or "perfume oil" as these types of oils will often have chemical or artificial ingredients added to them. Additives and adulteration (meaning adjusting or altering the oil in some way) have the potential to be harmful to the body and they also create weak, ineffective results in aromatherapy.

Quality
The quality of an essential oil is determined by a number of factors including;

♦ The plant species
♦ The quality of the soil
♦ The weather conditions/temperature
♦ Where the plants are grown – indoors/outdoors
♦ The extraction method used

The actual bottle of essential oil will not provide this information so this is where proper research comes into play. A reputable company should monitor the production of their oils from start to finish, and provide the general public with information on how they carry out this process. Always research the company's website and any literature they provide.

Price

The price of essential oil varies enormously and depends on how difficult or easy it is to extract the oil from the plant. For example, 2 million rose petals are needed to make just 1 ounce of Rose oil, making it one of the most expensive essential oils on the market. Alternatively it takes approximately 30kg of eucalyptus leaves to make 1 liter of Eucalyptus oil, making it one of the lesser expensive oils. When choosing, make sure the oils are not unusually cheap, especially the more expensive ones like Rose, Melissa, Neroli or Jasmine. This could mean they may not be pure or of good quality. It is a good idea to compare different brands to get an overall idea of how much your chosen essential oils should cost.

Storage

Essential oils are precious and expensive. It is therefore vital that they are stored correctly to ensure both their longevity and effectiveness. When you are purchasing oils or creating a blend at home, the following factors should be adhered to, to ensure you get the most from you oils;

> ➤ Make sure they are contained within dark amber or cobalt blue bottles. Sunlight can have a detrimental effect on the chemistry of essential oils causing them to deteriorate rapidly and lose their therapeutic benefits. Dark colored glass bottles offer protection from the sun's harmful ultra violet rays.

> ➤ Ensure the bottles are tightly sealed. Any prolonged contact with the air will cause essential oils to lose their composition and evaporate.

> ➤ Keep essential oils stored in a cool, dry place. Do not store them in an area where they will be subject to extreme changes in temperature. The heat will evaporate the oil whereas the cold will cause it to lose its composition.

> ➤ When purchasing essential or carrier oils, never buy oils that have dust on the cap or bottle. This is a sure sign that they have been sitting there for some time. Don't be afraid to ask the retailer when the oils arrived into the shop.

> ➤ Avoid aluminum or plastic bottles as the molecular structure of the oil will be affected.

Most essential oils have a shelf life of at least 2 years, particularly ones that have gone through steam distillation. There are some exceptions to this however, so make sure you do some research first (Tea Tree oil normally lasts for approximately 12 to 18 months). Citrus oils like Lemon, Orange, Bergamot, Mandarin or Neroli have the shortest shelf life of around 9 to 12 months.

It is important to note that carrier oils should be treated with as much careful consideration. They will go rancid very quickly if not stored properly. Most carrier oils have a shelf life of up to 2 years, with the exception of borage oil and flaxseed oil – these are very delicate and have a shelf life of about 6 months. Coconut and jojoba oils last for about 4 years and are often added to other carrier oils to extend the shelf life of a blend.

As you can see it is so important to take good care of your oils. Treating them with the love and attention they deserve will ensure they last longer, providing you with outstanding therapeutic benefits.

Use the following checklist as a guide when purchasing your essential oils:

Is the Latin name of the plant provided? This will ensure you are getting the correct variation of a particular oil, for example, there are several varieties of eucalyptus.
Where is the oil from? Sometimes quality can vary between countries.
What is the purity of the oil? It should be 100% essential oil. Avoid terms like "nature-identical", "fragrance oil" and "perfume oil".
Is the essential oil stored in a dark amber or cobalt blue glass container?
Are the bottles sealed tightly. If the seals have been broken, the oil could be compromised so avoid.
Where are the oils stored? Are they away from heaters or radiators? Are they away from direct sunlight?
How long has the oil been in stock?
How has the essential oil been extracted? This will give you an indication as to its shelf life.
Are the prices comparable to other brands? If they are unusually cheap, they could be dilutions so be careful.
Are the more expensive oils like Rose or Jasmine priced the same as say, Lemongrass or Rosemary? If so, they are more than likely diluted.

9
The Safety of Essential Oils

Used correctly, essential oils are very safe and can be used effectively to treat a number of specific conditions such as dry skin or insomnia. There is however, a possibility that oils used in the wrong dilutions or the overuse of any particular oil, may cause irritation and produce adverse effects. To prevent this from happening, there are several safety guidelines that should be followed, ensuring that you get the best from your blend.

❖ Allergy testing – before using an essential oil for the first time, particularly if you have sensitive skin or suffer from allergies, it is important you carry out a patch test on a small area of skin. To do this;

1. Blend 5ml of your chosen carrier oil along with 4 drops of essential oil, and apply to a small section on the inside of your elbow.
2. Apply a plaster or bandage over the area and leave for 24 hours.
3. If you encounter any symptoms such as itching, redness, inflammation, stinging or rash, remove the essential oil with cool, clean water.
4. If no irritation occurs after the 24 hour period, then you know it is safe to use.

Some carrier oils may contain traces of nut so it is imperative to avoid these oils if you suffer from nut allergies. Peanut and Hazelnut oils are obvious examples but all carrier oils should be checked before use.

❖ Skin irritants – while you may not have experienced any adverse reactions to the patch test, there are certain essential oils that can be irritating to the skin and should therefore be used with care. These include; *Basil, Benzoin, Black pepper, Cinnamon, Clove, Ginger, Lemon, Lemongrass, Melissa, Orange, Oregano, Peppermint, Pine, Thyme, Tea tree.*

❖ Medication – using essential oils while taking medication is not recommended as some oils can interfere with certain prescription medication. Always consult your doctor before using any oil.

- ❖ Photosensitivity – certain essential oils (mainly citrus oils) contain constituents that absorb sunlight/UV rays, increasing the effect sun can have on the skin. Using these oils before going out into the sun or using the sun bed can increase your chances of hyper pigmentation, sunburn, blisters or rash. The following oils should be avoided prior to UV exposure; *Bergamot, Lemon, Lemongrass, Mandarin, Orange, Lime, Grapefruit.*

- ❖ Avoid contact with the eyes. If any essential oil enters the eyes, rinse out immediately with plenty of cold water.

- ❖ Never use essential oils during the 1st trimester of pregnancy. For the remainder of the term, consult with your doctor before using any essential oils as most are not recommended.

- ❖ Never ingest essential oils unless it clearly states the nutritional content and instructions for use on the label.

- ❖ Essential oils should never be used on open cuts or wounds.

- ❖ With the vast number of essential oils available, there are some which should be completely avoided due to their toxicity. The following is a list of toxic oils which should never be used, under any circumstances;

Aniseed	Pennyroyal
Arnica	Rue
Bitter Almond	Sage
Boldo	Sassafras
Broom	Savin
Buchu	Savory
Calamus	Tansy
Camphor	Thuja
Cassia	Tonka
Horseradish	Wintergreen
Jaborandi	Wormseed
Mugwort	Wormwood

10
Aromatherapy for Beauty

Acne & Blemished Skin

Acne is a skin condition that is caused by the over production of oil in the sebaceous glands. This excess oil mixes with dead cells on the surface of the skin, causing the follicle to become blocked. Bacteria, that are already present on the skin, contaminate the follicle resulting in the appearance of blackheads, pimples, whiteheads, nodules or cysts.

The common treatments for acne are often prescribed antibiotics, harsh antibacterial face washes, and/or steroids. Over time, these can have a harmful effect on the skin, causing sensitization, facial swelling, redness, and irritation. As a result, many people turn to essential oils as an alternative holistic treatment, due to the powerful antibacterial and anti-inflammatory properties they possess.

Essential oils for acne & blemished skin; Benzoin, Bergamot, Cedarwood, Chamomile (German or Roman), Clary Sage, Geranium, Grapefruit, Juniper Berry, Lavender, Lemon, Lemongrass, Mandarin, Orange (Sweet), Rosemary, Tea Tree, Thyme.

Carrier oils for acne & blemished skin; Sweet Almond, Borage Seed, Coconut, Hazelnut.

❧ Facial Oils ❧

Blend all the ingredients together and mix thoroughly. Apply the formula to a cleansed face and neck, and gently massage using small circular movements. Leave the oils to absorb into the skin cells, do not wash off. Carry out the treatment twice per day, once in the morning and again at night. At night, a facial oil can be substituted with a facial moisturizer (recipes below) if you prefer. The following recipes will yield enough for 1 treatment. Where coconut oil is used in these recipes, make sure to use Raw Virgin Coconut Oil as it is the best form of coconut oil to use for the skin. Melt it by placing an even tablespoon into a cup, place the cup into a saucepan of boiling water, and continue to boil the water on the heat until the coconut oil has melted. Never melt in the microwave.

Day Blend 1
1 tablespoon coconut oil
5 drops of tea tree
4 drops of lavender
1 drop of geranium

Day Blend 2
1 tablespoon jojoba oil
10 drops of tea tree

Day Blend 3
1 tablespoon borage seed oil
4 drops of chamomile
4 drops of thyme
2 drops of lavender

Day Blend 4
1 tablespoon coconut oil
4 drops of lemon
4 drops of geranium
2 drops of neroli

Night Blend 1
1 tablespoon sweet almond oil
6 drops of bergamot
6 drops of tea tree
3 drops of lemon

Night Blend 2
1 tablespoon borage seed oil
10 drops of tea tree
5 drops of lavender

Night Blend 3
1 tablespoon coconut oil
10 drops of rosemary
2 drops of grapefruit
2 drops of juniper
1 drop of lavender

Night Blend 4
1 tablespoon jojoba oil
8 drops of lemongrass
4 drops of chamomile
3 drops of tea tree

❧ Facial Cleansers ❧

Blend all ingredients together and mix thoroughly. Apply the formula to the face and neck, and massage into the skin using outward circular movements. Leave to absorb into the skin for 2 minutes. Gently remove all traces of oil preferably using a wet muslin cloth soaked in warm water. A small, soft face towel can be used as an alternative. Repeat twice per day, once in the morning and again at night before applying a facial oil or moisturizer. The following recipes will yield enough for 1 treatment. Regarding coconut oil, please refer to 'Facial Oils' above for instructions on how to prepare.

Blend 1

1 tablespoon aloe vera gel
1 tablespoon coconut milk
8 drops of tea tree
4 drops of peppermint
2 drops of lavender

Blend 2

2 tablespoons raw honey
5 drops of rosemary
5 drops of lavender
5 drops of grapefruit

Blend 3

2 tablespoons extra virgin olive oil
4 drops of lemon
4 drops of grapefruit
2 drops of peppermint
2 drops of tea tree

Blend 4

1 tablespoon coconut milk
1 teaspoon coconut oil
15 drops of tea tree

❧ Facial Scrubs ❧

Combine all ingredients in a small bowl, mix thoroughly and use immediately. Massage the blend gently into the skin as you would the facial cleanser, paying particular attention to problem areas. Leave on the skin for 2 minutes and wash off with warm water. Carry out this treatment once per week. The following recipes will yield enough for 1 treatment. Regarding coconut oil, please refer to 'Facial Oils' above for instructions on how to prepare.

Blend 1
1 tablespoon baking soda
1 teaspoon water
10 drops of tea tree
2 drops of lavender
2 drops of chamomile

Blend 2
1 teaspoon brown sugar
6 drops of rosemary
5 drops of bergamot
2 drops of grapefruit
2 drops of geranium

Blend 3
½ cup ground oatmeal
1 tablespoon raw honey
1 teaspoon jojoba oil
6 drops of benzoin
6 drops of tea tree
6 drops of rosemary

Blend 4
1 teaspoon baking soda
1 teaspoon fresh lemon juice
1 teaspoon olive oil
4 drops of frankincense
4 drops of sandalwood
2 drops of lavender
2 drops of tea tree
2 drops of chamomile

❧ Facial Toners ❧

Blend all ingredients in a glass bottle and shake well to combine. You can use a spray bottle if you wish but it is not necessary. Always add the hydrosol (flower water) first and then follow with the essential oils. Distilled water is a great alternative to hydrosols but always ensure you use distilled water (tap water may contain chemicals or bacteria). If you are using a spray bottle, hold it 3 to 4 inches away from the face, close your eyes and spray. Do not wipe off. If you are using a normal bottle, soak a cotton pad with the toner and gently pat all over the face and neck. Apply each time after cleansing, exfoliating or a face mask. The following recipes will yield enough for approximately 2 to 3 days.

Blend 1
½ cup cold green tea
½ cup apple cider vinegar
10 drops of tea tree

Blend 2
1 cup distilled water
10 drops of rosemary
5 drops of bergamot

Blend 3
1 cup witch hazel
4 drops of geranium
4 drops of lemongrass
4 drops of tea tree

Blend 4
½ cup distilled water
Juice from 1 lemon
4 drops of grapefruit
4 drops of tea tree
4 drops of orange (sweet)
2 drops of peppermint

❧ Facial Moisturizers ❧

Blend all ingredients together and mix thoroughly. After cleansing and toning, apply the formula onto the face and neck, and massage into the skin, using small, gentle circular movements with the fingertips. If you are applying a day blend, allow the oils to absorb into the skin for 2 minutes before applying makeup. Repeat twice per day, once in the morning and again at night. A moisturizer may be substituted for a facial oil (recipes above) if you wish. The following recipes will yield enough for 1 – 2 treatments. Regarding coconut oil, please refer to 'Facial Oils' above for instructions on how to prepare.

Blend 1

5 tablespoons jojoba oil

7 tablespoons coconut oil

2 tablespoons aloe vera gel

* mix the above ingredients in a blender. Once blended, scoop out, and add;

15 drops of tea tree

5 drops of lavender

2 drops of chamomile

2 drops of bergamot

2 drops of rosemary

Blend 2

2 tablespoons shea butter

1 tablespoon rosehip seed oil

2 vitamin E capsules

*mix the above ingredients in a blender. Once blended, scoop out, and add;

8 drops of frankincense

8 drops of grapefruit

6 drops of sandalwood

2 drops of lavender

Blend 3

2 tablespoons aloe vera gel

4 tablespoons jojoba oil

Juice from ½ lemon

1 tablespoon coconut milk

*mix the above ingredients in a blender. Once blended, scoop out, and add;

20 drops of tea tree

Blend 4

½ cup distilled water

1 teaspoon fresh lemon juice

1 tablespoon extra virgin olive oil

1 tablespoon jojoba oil

mix the above ingredients in a blender. Once blended, scoop out, and add;

6 drops of lemon

6 drops of lavender

4 drops of grapefruit

2 drops of bergamot

❧ Facial Masks ❧

Blend all ingredients in a small bowl, mix thoroughly and use immediately. Apply the formula with either a mask brush or clean fingers, after the skin has been cleansed. Leave on for 15 to 20 minutes and wash off with warm water. Pat dry the face, follow with a toner and moisturizer or facial oil. Apply a face mask once every week. The following recipes will yield enough for 1 treatment.

Blend 1

2 tablespoons raw honey

1 tablespoon apple cider vinegar

4 drops of frankincense

4 drops of chamomile

4 drops of thyme

4 drops of tea tree

Blend 2

1 small ripe banana (mashed)

1 tablespoon raw honey

2 teaspoons fresh lemon juice

10 drops of tea tree

6 drops of chamomile

4 drops of clary sage

Blend 3

2 egg whites

Juice from ½ lemon

6 drops of benzoin

6 drops of bergamot

2 drops of cypress

2 drops of chamomile

Blend 4

4 tablespoons coconut oil

1 tablespoon raw honey

1 tablespoon baking soda

10 drops of chamomile

5 drops of lavender

Blend 5

2 tablespoons raw honey
1 teaspoon cinnamon
Juice from ¼ lemon
5 drops of thyme
5 drops of benzoin
5 drops of tea tree

Blend 6

2 tablespoons plain yogurt
1 tablespoon aloe vera gel
1 teaspoon jojoba oil
5 drops of tea tree
2 drops of bergamot
2 drops of grapefruit
2 drops of lavender

❧ Facial Spritz ❧

Blend all ingredients together in a spray bottle and mix thoroughly. Hold the bottle 3-4 inches from the face, close your eyes and spritz liberally. Repeat several times per day. The following recipes will yield enough for approximately 2 days.

Blend 1

50ml distilled water
15 drops of tea tree

Blend 2

50ml lavender hydrosol
5 drops of chamomile
5 drops of benzoin
5 drops of lavender

Blend 3

50ml distilled water
2 tablespoons aloe vera juice
10 drops of bergamot
5 drops of rosemary

Blend 4

50ml distilled water
1 tablespoon apple cider vinegar
1 tablespoon fresh lemon juice
2 drops of geranium
2 drops of clary sage
2 drops of chamomile
2 drops of juniper berry

❧ Topical Treatments ❧

Tea tree and lavender are the only 2 essential oils recommended for direct use on blemishes. It is always advised to apply with a cotton bud as bacteria may be present on the fingertips. If you do not have cotton buds to hand, make sure and wash your hands thoroughly before application. Once applied, there is no need to wash off. Essential oils can cause irritation to the skin if overused, particularly tea tree in undiluted form, therefore topical treatments should only be carried out 2-4 times per week.

Blend 1
Apply 2 drops of tea tree on a cotton bud and gently tap the pimple.

Blend 2
Apply 1 drop of lavender and 1 drop of tea tree on a cotton bud and gently tap the pimple.

Age Spots

Age spots, also known as brown spots or liver spots, are flat, brown areas of pigmentation that vary in size and usually appear on the face, hand, neck, arms and shoulders. They are caused by excessive exposure to the sun, and while they are very common in maturing adults, they can affect younger people as well. Over time, essential oils can lighten age spots and in some cases completely remove them.

Essential oils for age spots; Cypress, Frankincense, Geranium, Grapefruit, Lavender, Lemon, Myrrh, Sandalwood, Ylang Ylang.

Carrier oils for age spots; Coconut (raw virgin), Evening Primrose, Jojoba.

❧ Massage Oils ❧

Blend all ingredients together and mix thoroughly. Apply to the age spot, or if there is a cluster of them, apply to the whole area. Leave to absorb into the skin, do not wash off. Repeat daily. The following recipes provide treatments for 1 week.

Blend 1
1 tablespoon raw virgin coconut oil
5 drops of myrrh
5 drops of frankincense
5 drops of lavender
*melt the coconut oil first, add essential oils and leave to solidify.

Blend 2
2 tablespoons jojoba oil
10 drops of frankincense
5 drops of sandalwood

Blend 3
1 tablespoon aloe vera gel
10 drops of sandalwood
2 drops of lemon
2 drops of cypress
1 drop of lavender

Blend 4
1 tablespoon raw virgin coconut oil
8 drops of frankincense
4 drops of geranium
2 drops of grapefruit
1 drop of ylang ylang

Aging/Mature Skin

Believe it or not the skin of individuals aged over 25 years is termed mature skin. Once we hit our mid twenties, collagen and elastin (proteins that keep the skin firm and supple) production in our skin cells starts to slow down. As a result the skin starts to develop signs of aging, including loss of elasticity, the appearance of fine lines and wrinkles, reduced muscle tone, thinner skin, and age spots, dilated capillaries and skin tags become more apparent. While these changes in the skin are a natural part of aging, essential oils help to slow down the aging process, keeping the skin looking younger and healthier for longer.

Essential oils for aging/mature skin; Frankincense, Geranium, Jasmine, Lavender, Myrrh, Neroli, Patchouli, Sandalwood, Rose, Rosewood.

Carrier oils for aging/mature skin; Sweet Almond, Avocado, Coconut (raw virgin), Evening Primrose, Jojoba, Rosehip Seed (not really a carrier oil as such but a fantastic nourishing and regenerating oil for the skin).

❧ Facial Oils ❧

Blend all the ingredients together and mix thoroughly. Apply the formula to a cleansed face and neck, and gently massage using small circular movements. Leave the oils to absorb into the skin cells, do not wash off. Carry out the treatment twice per day, once in the morning and again at night. At night, a facial oil can be substituted with a facial moisturizer (recipes below) if you prefer. The following recipes will yield enough for 1 treatment. Where coconut oil is used in these recipes, make sure to use Raw Virgin Coconut Oil as it is the best form of coconut oil to use for the skin. Melt it by placing an even tablespoon into a cup, place the cup into a saucepan of boiling water, and continue to boil the water on the heat until the coconut oil has melted. Never melt in the microwave.

Blend 1

2 tablespoons melted coconut oil
6 drops of frankincense
5 drops of geranium
2 drops of neroli
2 drops of rose

Blend 2

2 tablespoons jojoba oil
6 drops of myrrh
6 drops of sandalwood
3 drops of jasmine

Blend 3

1 tablespoon avocado oil
1 teaspoon rosehip seed oil
5 drops of frankincense
5 drops of myrrh
3 drops of sandalwood
2 drops of lavender

Blend 4

1 tablespoon melted coconut oil
1 teaspoon rosehip seed oil
6 drops of neroli
4 drops of rose
4 drops of frankincense
1 drop of jasmine

❧ Facial Cleansers ❧

Blend all ingredients together and mix thoroughly. Apply the formula to the face and neck, and massage into the skin using outward circular movements. Leave to absorb into the skin for 2 minutes. Gently remove all traces of oil preferably using a wet muslin cloth soaked in warm water. A small, soft face towel can be used as an alternative. Repeat twice per day, once in the morning and again at night before applying a facial oil or moisturizer. The following recipes will yield enough for 1 treatment. Regarding coconut oil, please refer to 'Facial Oils' above for instructions on how to prepare.

Blend 1

1 tablespoon jojoba oil
1 teaspoon melted coconut oil (raw virgin)
6 drops of carrot seed
6 drops of frankincense
3 drops of sandalwood

Blend 2

1 tablespoon aloe vera gel
1 vitamin E capsule
5 drops of jasmine
5 drops of rosemary
5 drops of lavender

Blend 3

1 tablespoon evening primrose
1 tablespoon melted coconut oil
8 drops of lavender
2 drops of geranium
2 drops of carrot seed
2 drops of myrrh
1 drop of rose

Blend 4

1 tablespoon melted cocoa butter
1 teaspoon rosehip seed oil
6 drops of clary sage
4 drops of lemon
4 drops of geranium
1 drop of neroli

❧ Facial Scrubs ❧

Combine all ingredients in a small bowl, mix thoroughly and use immediately. Massage the blend gently into the skin as you would the facial cleanser. Leave on the skin for 2 minutes and wash off with warm water. Carry out this treatment once per week. The following recipes will yield enough for 1 treatment. Regarding coconut oil, please refer to 'Facial Oils' above for instructions on how to prepare.

Blend 1
1 tablespoon plain natural yogurt
1 teaspoon ground oatmeal
1 teaspoon melted coconut oil
5 drops of jasmine
2 drops of myrrh
1 drop of patchouli

Blend 2
1 tablespoon ground oatmeal
1 tablespoon coconut milk
1 vitamin E capsule
4 drops of chamomile
4 drops of frankincense

Blend 3
1 tablespoon mashed papaya
1 teaspoon manuka honey
6 drops of frankincense
2 drops of lavender

Blend 4
1 tablespoon manuka honey
1 teaspoon ground almond meal
4 drops of rosemary
3 drops of geranium
1 drop of neroli

❧ Facial Toners ❧

Blend all ingredients in a glass bottle and shake well to combine. You can use a spray bottle if you wish but it is not necessary. Always add the hydrosol (flower water) first and then follow with the essential oils. Distilled water is a great alternative to hydrosols but always ensure you use distilled water (tap water may contain chemicals or bacteria). If you are using a spray bottle, hold it 3 to 4 inches away from the face, close your eyes and spray. Do not wipe off. If you are using a normal bottle, soak a cotton pad with the toner and gently pat all over the face and neck. Apply each time after cleansing, exfoliating or a face mask. The following recipes will yield enough for approximately 2 to 3 days.

Blend 1
50ml distilled water
10 drops of lavender
5 drops of rosewood
5 drops of jasmine
5 drops of patchouli

Blend 2
50ml rose water
20ml aloe vera juice
10 drops of frankincense
10 drops of rose
5 drops of geranium

Blend 3
50ml distilled water
10 drops of frankincense
10 drops of geranium

Blend 4
50ml rose water
15 drops of rose
10 drops of neroli

❧ Facial Masks ❧

Blend all ingredients in a small bowl, mix thoroughly and use immediately. Apply the formula with either a mask brush or clean fingers, after the skin has been cleansed. Leave on for 15 to 20 minutes and wash off with warm water. Pat dry the face, follow with a toner and moisturizer or facial oil. Apply a face mask once every week. The following recipes will yield enough for 1 treatment.

Blend 1

½ ripe avocado, mashed
1 teaspoon rosehip seed oil
5 drops of frankincense
5 drops of rosemary
5 drops of myrrh

Blend 2

1 tablespoon manuka honey
1 tablespoon evening primrose oil
8 drops of carrot seed
4 drops of sandalwood
3 drops of rose

Blend 3

1 tablespoon cocoa powder
1 vitamin E capsule
1 teaspoon coconut milk
1 teaspoon rosehip seed oil
Mix into a paste and then add;
6 drops of clary sage
4 drops of rosemary
3 drops of geranium
2 drops of lavender

Blend 4

1 tablespoon aloe vera gel
1 teaspoon avocado oil
1 teaspoon jojoba oil
6 drops of jasmine
6 drops of cedarwood
2 drops of neroli
1 drop of lavender

❧ Facial Moisturizers ❧

Blend all ingredients together and mix thoroughly. After cleansing and toning, apply the formula onto the face and neck, and massage into the skin, using small, gentle circular movements with the fingertips. If you are applying a day blend, allow the oils to absorb into the skin for 2 minutes before applying makeup. Repeat twice per day, once in the morning and again at night. A moisturizer may be substituted for a facial oil (recipes above) if you wish. The following recipes will yield enough for 1 – 2 treatments. Regarding coconut oil, please refer to 'Facial Oils' above for instructions on how to prepare.

Blend 1

1 tablespoon vegetable glycerin
1 teaspoon aloe vera gel
1 teaspoon rose water
8 drops of rose
4 drops of neroli
3 drops of lavender

Blend 2

1 tablespoon shea butter
2 vitamin E capsules
1 teaspoon rosehip seed oil
Mix the above ingredients in a blender. Once blended, scoop out and add;
10 drops of frankincense
5 drops of sandalwood

Blend 3

1 tablespoon melted beeswax
1 teaspoon melted coconut oil
1 teaspoon rosehip seed oil
6 drops of neroli
6 drops of jasmine
3 drops of rose
Allow the formula to solidify once all ingredients have been added.

Blend 4

1 tablespoons melted coconut oil
5 drops of geranium
5 drops of myrrh
5 drops of sandalwood

Cellulite

Cellulite is the buildup of fat, water and waste deposits under the skin, giving it a dimpled, lumpy appearance. It is a very frustrating condition and can be a major cause of misery for a lot of women. Thankfully essential oils can be a very effective remedy, when included with a healthy diet and exercise regime.

Essential oils for cellulite; Benzoin, Cedarwood, Cypress, Fennel, Geranium, Grapefruit, Juniper, Lemon, Mandarin, Orange, Rosemary, Thyme.

Carrier oils for cellulite; Sweet Almond Oil, Coconut Oil, Jojoba Oil.

Anti Cellulite Plan (repeat daily)

➢ Begin by dry brushing the entire body, using light upward strokes (always brush in the direction of the heart).

➢ Have a warm to hot bath using the cellulite bath blends. Soak for 20 minutes. While soaking, pinch and deeply massage areas of cellulite to help break down fatty deposits.

➢ Immediately after the bath (pores will be open), apply a cellulite massage blend to the entire affected limb, for example, if you suffer from cellulite on the top of your legs, massage the entire leg and buttocks area. This will disperse the toxins and improve the flow of blood.

➢ Drink 2 liters of water each day. This encourages the elimination of toxins.

➢ Do exercises that work specifically on the affected area.

➢ Use a cellulite body scrub and apply a cellulite body wrap 2–3 times per week.

❧ Massage Oils ❧

Blend all ingredients together and mix thoroughly. Apply to the affected limb. When massaging, firmly grip the tissue, lifting it away from the muscles underneath. Using a kneading motion with your knuckles, rub the entire affected area as firmly as you can. Take care not to cause bruising but don't be afraid to massage firmly. Repeat daily. The following recipes will yield enough for 1 treatment.

Blend 1
2 tablespoons sweet almond oil
6 drops of benzoin
6 drops of rosemary
6 drops of cypress
6 drops of cedarwood

Blend 2
2 tablespoons coconut oil
6 drops of rosemary
6 drops of grapefruit
6 drops of fennel
6 drops of juniper

Blend 3
2 tablespoons sweet almond oil
10ml jojoba oil
6 drops of rosemary
6 drops of grapefruit
6 drops of thyme
6 drops of lemon

Blend 4
2 tablespoons sweet almond oil
6 drops of juniper
6 drops of mandarin
6 drops of geranium
6 drops of cedarwood

Blend 5
2 tablespoons coconut oil
10 drops of grapefruit
10 drops of rosemary

Blend 6
2 tablespoons jojoba oil
6 drops of thyme
6 drops of fennel
6 drops of juniper
6 drops of lemon

❧ Body Scrubs ❧

A body scrub can not only help lessen the appearance of cellulite, it also exfoliates the skin and improves circulation. This improved circulation will help to loosen up excess fluid and eliminate toxins at a quicker rate.

Place all ingredients in a small bowl and mix thoroughly. Before a shower/bath, lather the scrub onto the affected area and massage into the skin using small, circular movements. Rinse off in the shower/bath and follow with a cellulite massage blend. Repeat 2-3 times per week. The following recipes will yield enough for 1 treatment.

Blend 1
½ cup ground coffee
½ cup brown sugar
2 tablespoons jojoba oil
10 drops of grapefruit
10 drops of rosemary

Blend 2
1 cup sea salt
2 tablespoons coconut oil
8 drops of fennel
8 drops of thyme
8 drops of benzoin
8 drops of lemon

Blend 3
½ cup brown sugar
½ cup sea salt
1 tablespoon sweet almond oil
6 drops of grapefruit
6 drops of orange
6 drops of geranium
6 drops of juniper

Blend 4
1 cup ground oatmeal
2 tablespoons jojoba oil
5 drops of cedarwood
5 drops of cypress
5 drops of thyme
5 drops of mandarin

❧ Bath Blends ❧

A warm Epsom salt bath with essential oils is a great addition to your anti-cellulite regime. It helps to eliminate toxins from the body, while the essential oils absorb into the bloodstream, boosting circulation and stimulating lymph flow. Always add the Epsom salts before running the water, make sure the water is warm and not hot. Add the essential oils to the bath water and agitate the water to disperse the oils. While in the bath, firmly massage the affected area using circular knuckling movements. Soak for 20 minutes. Repeat daily. Drink 2 glasses of water after the bath.

Blend 1
2 cups Epsom salts
3 drops of juniper
3 drops of fennel
3 drops of cypress
3 drops of grapefruit

Blend 2
2 cups Epsom salts
5 drops of rosemary
5 drops of benzoin
3 drops of lemon

Blend 3
2 cups Epsom salts
15 drops of grapefruit

Blend 4
2 cups Epsom salts
5 drops of geranium
5 drops of orange
5 drops of lemon

❧ Body Wraps ❧

Body wraps are designed to improve the texture and appearance of the skin by helping to rid the body of excess fluids and toxins. They are a fantastic way to help with cellulite and have many positive benefits including detoxification, skin tightening, skin softening and temporary inch loss.

To apply a body wrap;

➤ Blend all ingredients in a small bowl and mix thoroughly. Apply the formula over the affected area.

➤ You can cover the formula using either a roll of cling film or large rolls of elastic bandages (you will need 12-20 depending on the size of the area being treated).

➤ Begin by wrapping at the bottom of the area in question. Wrap tightly but not so tight as to cut off circulation.

➤ You can use a safety pin to hold the wraps in place but simply tucking the end of the bandage into the wrap itself will be sufficient.

➤ Do not expose any area of skin.

➤ Leave the wrap on for 30-45 minutes and during that time, drink 2 glasses of water.

➤ Depending on the ingredients used (for e.g., clay, coffee or manuka honey) you may need to have a shower afterwards. For simple aromatherapy oil blends, a shower is not necessary.

Blend 1
5 tablespoons aloe vera gel
15 drops of grapefruit
5 drops of cypress

Blend 2
½ cup extra virgin olive oil
5 drops of benzoin
5 drops of fennel
5 drops of lemon
5 drops of juniper

Blend 3
5 tablespoons manuka honey
5 tablespoons lemon juice
5 drops of grapefruit
5 drops of fennel
5 drops of juniper

Blend 4
½ cup coconut oil
4 tablespoons grapefruit juice
1 teaspoon baking soda
10 drops of rosemary
5 drops of lemon
5 drops of cypress

Blend 5

½ cup coconut oil
1 tablespoon lemon juice
10 drops of rosemary
10 drops of cedarwood
10 drops of geranium

Blend 6

½ cup ground coffee
½ cup sea salt
Juice of 1 lemon
5 drops of thyme
5 drops of cypress
5 drops of rosemary

Suggested daily cellulite regime using essential oils;

♦ Dry Brushing
♦ Warm bath
♦ Massage oils

Suggested cellulite regime – 2 to 3 times per week;

♦ Body scrub
♦ Warm bath
♦ Body wrap
♦ Massage oils

Chapped Lips

Because our lips do not contain oil glands, they are prone to dryness and chapping if not protected from the elements. Essential oils make for easy-to-make natural lip remedies.

Essential oils for chapped lips; Chamomile (Roman), Eucalyptus, Frankincense, Geranium, Neroli, Peppermint, Rose, Sandalwood, Tea Tree.

Carrier oils for chapped lips; Aloe Vera Gel (not a carrier oil but an effective treatment for chapped lips), Sweet Almond, Coconut, Rosehip.

❧ Massage Oils ❧

Blend all ingredients together and mix thoroughly. Apply to lips. Leave to absorb, do not wash off. Repeat 2-3 times per day. The following recipes will make treatments for 1 day, apart from blend 4, this should last approximately 2-3 days.

Blend 1
1 teaspoon aloe vera gel
2 drops of chamomile
2 drops of eucalyptus

Blend 2
1 teaspoon aloe vera gel
3 drops of peppermint
1 drop of geranium

Blend 3
1 tablespoon extra virgin olive oil
2 lavender
2 geranium

Blend 4
1 tablespoon beeswax pellets
1 tablespoon raw virgin coconut oil
2 vitamin E capsules
1 drop of frankincense
1 drops of lavender
1 drop of geranium
1 drop of peppermint

melt the beeswax and coconut oil, add the essential oils and vitamin E capsule and leave to solidify.

Dilated Capillaries

Also known as broken capillaries or facial thread veins, this condition usually affect fair-skinned people and is the result of poor circulation or the loss of elasticity in capillary walls. Certain essential oils help to reduce vascularity, restore some elasticity to the blood vessels, and increase circulation.

Essential oils for dilated capillaries; Chamomile (Roman), Cypress, Geranium, Lemon, Neroli, Rose.

Carrier oils for dilated capillaries; Sweet Almond, Argan, Avocado, Borage Seed, Coconut, Evening Primrose, Wheatgerm.

❧ Massage Oils ❧

Blend all ingredients together and mix thoroughly. Very gently massage the formula into the area in question. Leave to absorb into the skin, do not wash off. Repeat daily.

Blend 1
1 tablespoon argan oil
1 teaspoon evening primrose oil
10 drops of chamomile
5 drops of rose

Blend 2
1 tablespoon coconut oil
5 drops of cypress
5 drops of neroli
5 drops of geranium

Blend 3
1 tablespoon sweet almond oil
8 drops of rosemary
7 drops of chamomile

Blend 4
1 tablespoon wheatgerm oil
10ml borage seed oil
8 drops of cypress
5 drops of geranium
2 drops of neroli

Dry Skin

Dry skin is a common condition and occurs when the skin lacks either oil or moisture. It has the following characteristics;

♦ Small & tight pores
♦ Coarse and thin skin texture
♦ Uneven skin pigmentation
♦ Broken capillaries and premature ageing is common
♦ Patches of flaky skin may appear

When choosing essential oils for dry skin, choose oils that help to regenerate skin cells, reduce inflammation, balance the production of oil and help to reduce skin ageing.

Essential oils for dry skin include; Benzoin, Chamomile German, Frankincense, Geranium, Lavender, Myrrh, Neroli, Palmarosa, Patchouli, Rosemary, Rosewood, Sandalwood.

Carrier oils for dry skin include; Almond, Apricot Kernel, Avocado, Coconut, Evening Primrose, Jojoba, Macadamia, Peach Kernel.

❧ Facial Oils ❧

Blend all the ingredients together and mix thoroughly. Apply the formula to a cleansed face and neck, and gently massage using small circular movements. Leave the oils to absorb into the skin cells, do not wash off. Carry out the treatment twice per day, once in the morning and again at night. At night, a facial oil can be substituted with a facial moisturizer (recipes below) if you prefer. The following recipes will yield enough for 1 treatment. Where coconut oil is used in these recipes, make sure to use Raw Virgin Coconut Oil as it is the best form of coconut oil to use for the skin. Melt it by placing an even tablespoon into a cup, place the cup into a saucepan of boiling water, and continue to boil the water on the heat until the coconut oil has melted. Never melt in the microwave.

Blend 1
1 tablespoon almond oil
8 drops of patchouli
4 drops of sandalwood
4 drops of myrrh

Blend 2
1 tablespoon jojoba oil
7 drops of palmarosa
5 drops of rosemary
4 drops of sandalwood

Blend 3

1 tablespoon apricot kernel oil
6 drops of lavender
4 drops of chamomile
4 drops of geranium
2 drops of myrrh

Blend 4

1 tablespoon coconut oil
8 drops of frankincense
8 drops of myrrh

❧ Facial Cleansers ❧

Blend all ingredients together and mix thoroughly. Apply the formula to the face and neck, and massage into the skin using outward circular movements. Leave to absorb into the skin for 2 minutes. Gently remove all traces of oil preferably using a wet muslin cloth soaked in warm water. A small, soft face towel can be used as an alternative. Repeat twice per day, once in the morning and again at night before applying a facial oil or moisturizer. The following recipes will yield enough for 1 treatment. Regarding coconut oil, please refer to 'Facial Oils' above for instructions on how to prepare.

Blend 1

1 tablespoon coconut oil
9 drops of lavender
6 drops of geranium

Blend 2

1 tablespoon extra virgin olive oil
6 drops of chamomile
6 drops of frankincense

Blend 3

1 tablespoon sweet almond oil
5 drops of palmarosa
2 drops of rosemary
2 drops of lavender

Blend 4

1 tablespoon macadamia oil
6 drops of sandalwood
2 drops of patchouli

❧ Facial Toners ❧

Blend all ingredients in a glass bottle and shake well to combine. You can use a spray bottle if you wish but it is not necessary. Always add the hydrosol (flower water) first and then follow with the essential oils. Distilled water is a great alternative to hydrosols but always ensure you use distilled water (tap water may contain chemicals or bacteria). If you are using a spray bottle, hold it 3 to 4 inches away from the face, close your eyes and spray. Do not wipe off. If you are using a normal bottle, soak a cotton pad with the toner and gently pat all over the face and neck. Apply each time after cleansing, exfoliating or a face mask. The following recipes will yield enough for approximately 2 to 3 days.

Blend 1
50ml rose water
5 drops of lavender
5 drops of chamomile
5 drops of sandalwood

Blend 2
40ml lavender water
10ml distilled water
10 drops of geranium
10 drops of bergamot

Blend 3
1 teaspoon witch hazel
40ml aloe vera juice
5 drops of palmarosa
5 drops of rosewood
2 drops of chamomile

Blend 4
50ml rose water
15 drops of rosemary

❧ Facial Moisturizers ❧

Blend all ingredients together and mix thoroughly. After cleansing and toning, apply the formula onto the face and neck, and massage into the skin, using small, gentle circular movements with the fingertips. If you are applying a day blend, allow the oils to absorb into the skin for 2 minutes before applying makeup. Repeat twice per day, once in the morning and again at night. A moisturizer may be substituted for a facial oil (recipes above) if you wish. The following recipes will yield enough for 1 – 2 treatments. Regarding coconut oil, please refer to 'Facial Oils' above for instructions on how to prepare.

Day Blend 1
1 tablespoon sweet almond oil
1 teaspoon jojoba oil
2 drops of lavender
2 drops of geranium
2 drops of ylang ylang

Day Blend 2
1 tablespoon coconut oil
6 drops of carrot seed
4 drops of myrrh
2 drops of frankincense
1 drop of lavender

Night Blend 1
1 tablespoon avocado oil
1 teaspoon vitamin E oil (1 capsule)
2 drops of rose
2 drops of neroli
2 drops of sandalwood

Night Blend 2
1 tablespoon rosehip seed oil
4 drops of frankincense
4 drops of myrrh

❧ Facial Scrubs ❧

Combine all ingredients in a small bowl, mix thoroughly and use immediately. Massage the blend gently into the skin as you would the facial cleanser. Leave on the skin for 2 minutes and wash off with warm water. Carry out this treatment once per week. The following recipes will yield enough for 1 treatment. Regarding coconut oil, please refer to 'Facial Oils' above for instructions on how to prepare.

Blend 1
1 cup of ground oatmeal
4 tablespoons of avocado oil
8 drops of patchouli
4 drops of ylang ylang
4 drops of chamomile

Blend 2
2 large tablespoons of manuka honey
½ cup of brown sugar
1 tablespoon of extra virgin olive oil
2 drops of geranium
2 drops of bergamot
1 drop of lavender

❧ Facial Masks ❧

Blend all ingredients in a small bowl, mix thoroughly and use immediately. Apply the formula with either a mask brush or clean fingers, after the skin has been cleansed. Leave on for 15 to 20 minutes and wash off with warm water. Pat dry the face, follow with a toner and moisturizer or facial oil. Apply a face mask once every week. The following recipes will yield enough for 1 treatment.

Blend 1
1 ripe avocado (mashed)
1 tablespoon of coconut oil
8 drops of frankincense
4 drops of myrrh
2 drops of chamomile

Blend 2
2 tablespoons of manuka honey
4 drops of ylang ylang
2 drops of geranium
2 drops of sandalwood

Blend 3
3 tablespoons of aloe vera gel
½ teaspoon of jojoba oil
6 drops of lavender
2 drops of palmarosa
2 drops of rosemary

Blend 4
2 tablespoons of unflavored yogurt
6 drops of neroli
4 drops of chamomile

❧ Facial Sauna ❧

Fill a large bowl with boiling water, add the chosen essential oils, place a towel around your head and lean towards the water (closing off the sides with the towel). The steam can burn your skin so hold your head as close as is comfortable. Close eyes and inhale deeply for 7 – 10 minutes.

Blend 1
1 large bowl of boiling water
8 drops of sandalwood

Blend 2
1 large bowl of boiling water
3 drops of lavender
3 drops of geranium
2 drops of frankincense

Hair Care

Essential oils can work wonders for the hair, whether you want to treat a dry, flaky scalp, stimulate hair growth, strengthen hair or improve condition. Choose from one of the following categories below and follow the recipes regularly for healthy, shiny hair.

Dandruff

Dandruff is a common dry scalp condition which causes flaking of the scalp and itching. It can be a very embarrassing and frustrating condition for some people but thankfully essential oils are a very effective way to treat and alleviate the problem.

Essential oils for dandruff; Basil, Cypress, Lavender, Lemon, Peppermint, Rosemary, Tea Tree, Thyme.

Carrier oils for dandruff; Borage Seed, Coconut, Evening Primrose, Jojoba.

❧ Massage Oils ❧

Blend all ingredients together and mix thoroughly. Pour a small amount into the palm of your hand and gently rub both hands together to evenly spread the formula. Massage it into the scalp, starting at the top of the forehead. Continue to apply the blend to the entire scalp until the oils have been used up. For 5 minutes, gently massage the scalp using the pads of the fingers in small, circular movements. Keep the blend on overnight or for as long as you can. Rinse and condition the hair as normal (add several drops of the same essential oils to your shampoo to boost results). Repeat 2-3 times per week. The following recipes will make 1 treatment.

Blend 1
1 tablespoon jojoba oil
1 tablespoon evening primrose oil
5 drops of rosemary
5 drops of lavender
5 drops of peppermint

Blend 2
2 tablespoons coconut oil
15 drops of tea tree

Blend 3

2 tablespoons jojoba oil
6 drops of basil
4 drops of lemon
3 drops of rosemary
2 drops of thyme

Blend 4

2 tablespoons macadamia oil
10 drops of tea tree
5 drops of rosemary

❧ Hair Rinse ❧

Blend all ingredients together and mix thoroughly. Massage into your scalp after shampooing/rinsing your hair. Leave for 5 minutes and rinse. Condition and style as normal. Repeat 2-3 times per week. The following recipes will make 1 treatment.

Blend 1

½ cup apple cider vinegar
10 drops of peppermint
5 drops of tea tree
5 drops of lavender

Blend 2

½ cup witch hazel
10 drops of tea tree
10 drops of rosemary

Dry, Damaged or Frizzy Hair

Dry hair is caused by the underproduction of oil glands in the scalp which results in the hair becoming dry, brittle and tangled. It can be further aggravated by the use of bleaching, tinting and regular hair coloring. Regular treatments using essential oils can nourish the scalp, rebalance oil production and condition and soften the hair.

Essential oils for dry, damaged or frizzy hair; Geranium, Lavender, Palmarosa, Rosemary, Sandalwood.

Carrier oils for dry, damaged or frizzy hair; Coconut, Jojoba, Macadamia, Olive, Peach Kernel.

❧ Massage Oils ❧

Blend all ingredients together and mix thoroughly. Pour a small amount into the palm of your hands and massage it into the scalp (add more oil if your hair is longer or thicker). Apply the remaining formula throughout the hair, making sure to cover the ends. Gently massage the scalp using small, circular movements for about 5 minutes. Leave on for several hours or overnight if you can (remember to protect your bed sheets). Rinse the treatment out thoroughly and condition your hair as normal. Repeat 2-3 times per week for the best results. Each of the following recipes carries out 1 treatment.

Blend 1
3 tablespoons jojoba oil
10 drops of lavender
5 drops of sandalwood

Blend 2
2 tablespoons extra virgin olive oil
5 drops of sandalwood
5 drops of palmarosa
5 drops of lavender
5 drops of rosemary
5 drops of geranium

Blend 3
3 tablespoons macadamia oil
10 drops of sandalwood
10 drops of lavender
5 drops of rosemary

Blend 4
2 tablespoons coconut oil
25 drops of lavender

❧ Treatment Shampoo ❧

Blend all ingredients together in a bowl and mix thoroughly. Apply to wet hair and massage into the scalp and hair. You may need to include more base shampoo depending on the length and thickness of your hair. The following formulas are for 1 treatment on medium length hair.

Blend 1

2 tablespoons unscented natural shampoo
1 vitamin E capsules
1 teaspoon jojoba oil
5 drops of sandalwood
5 drops of geranium

Blend 2

2 tablespoons unscented natural shampoo
1 teaspoon macadamia oil
5 drops of lavender
5 drops of palmarosa

❧ Treatment Masks ❧

Adding a mask treatment to your healthy hair regime can really boost results by helping to further condition, nourish and improve the texture of hair. Blend all ingredients in a small bowl and mix thoroughly. Apply to damp, clean hair. Divide the hair into section and massage the mask into the hair and scalp, paying particular attention to the ends. Leave on for 1 hour and thoroughly rinse and condition hair as normal. Repeat twice per week. Each of the following recipes are for 1 treatment on medium length hair.

Blend 1

2 tablespoons coconut milk
1 tablespoon raw, unprocessed honey
2 tablespoons extra virgin olive oil
10 drops of lavender
5 drops of sandalwood

Blend 2

½ ripe avocado (mashed)
1 tablespoon jojoba oil
1 tablespoon macadamia oil
5 drops of rosemary
5 drops of palmarosa
5 drops of geranium

Hair Lice

Lice are parasites that infest the hair and must be dealt with immediately as they can spread by direct contact. Compared to traditional pharmaceutical treatments, essential oils are a non-toxic, safe alternative for eliminating head lice as they can effectively kill lice and their eggs.

Essential oils for head lice; Eucalyptus, Geranium, Lavender, Lavender, Lemon, Rosemary, Tea Tree, Thyme.

Carrier oils for head lice; Sweet Almond, Coconut, Evening Primrose, Grapeseed, Jojoba.

❧ Massage Oils ❧

Blend all ingredients together and mix thoroughly. Wash, (shampoo with added drops of tea tree will boost results), towel dry and meticulously comb the hair. Vigorously massage the formula into the scalp, ensuring that the entire scalp is covered. Leave the treatment on for 2-3 hours and rinse. Repeat each night until the lice have been eliminated. The following recipes will make 1 treatment.

Blend 1
3 tablespoons coconut oil
15 drops of tea tree
10 drops of lavender
5 drops of rosemary

Blend 2
3 tablespoons jojoba oil
10 drops of rosemary
10 drops of geranium
10 drops of lavender

Blend 3
3 tablespoons grapeseed oil
10 drops of eucalyptus
10 drops of rosemary
5 drops of lemon
5 drops of lavender

Blend 4
3 tablespoons coconut oil
10 drops of lemon
10 drops of tea tree
10 drops of thyme

Hair Loss & Regrowth

The most important factor to consider when treating any kind of hair loss is a healthy scalp. Massaging the scalp regularly with certain essential oils stimulates the blood vessels of the scalp to send vital nutrients and oxygen to the hair follicles at a faster rate. Over time, this encourages growth and improves the condition and texture of hair.

Essential oils for hair loss & regrowth; Cedarwood, Chamomile (Roman), Clary Sage, Cypress, Lavender, Lemon, Rosemary, Thyme.

Carrier oils for hair loss & regrowth; Coconut, Evening Primrose, Grapeseed, Jojoba.

❧ Massage Oils ❧

Blend all ingredients together and mix thoroughly. Pour a small amount into the palm of your hand and gently rub both hands together to evenly spread the formula. Massage it into the scalp, starting at the top of the forehead. Continue to apply the blend to the entire scalp until the oils have been used up. For 5 minutes, gently massage the scalp using the pads of the fingers in small, circular movements. Keep the blend on overnight or for as long as you can. Rinse and condition the hair as normal (add several drops of the same essential oils to your shampoo to boost results). Repeat 2-3 times per week. The following recipes will make 1 treatment.

Blend 1
2 tablespoons grapeseed
1 teaspoon jojoba oil
5 drops of lavender
5 drops of thyme
5 drops of rosemary

Blend 2
2 tablespoons evening primrose oil
8 drops of rosemary
7 drops of thyme

Blend 3
1 tablespoon jojoba oil
1 tablespoon macadamia oil
5 drops of thyme
5 drops of cedarwood
5 drops of clary sage

Blend 4
1 tablespoon coconut oil
1 tablespoon evening primrose oil
6 drops of rosemary
4 drops of lavender
2 drops of cypress
2 drops of chamomile
1 drop of lemon

Oily Hair

Oily hair is the result of the overproduction of oil glands in the scalp. Hair is characteristically limp and lifeless, and can look greasy. Shampoo with harsh chemicals and detergents can often worsen the problem as they stimulate excess oil production, so including more natural products in your hair care regime is recommended.

Essential oils for oily hair; Cypress, Grapefruit, Juniper Berry, Lavender, Lemon, Peppermint, Rosemary.

Carrier oils for oily hair; Sweet Almond, Coconut, Grapeseed, Jojoba.

❧ Massage Oils ❧

Blend all ingredients together and mix thoroughly. Pour a small amount into the palm of your hands and massage it into the scalp (add more oil if your hair is longer or thicker). Apply the remaining formula throughout the hair, making sure to cover the ends. Gently massage the scalp using small, circular movements for about 5 minutes. Leave on for several hours or overnight if you can (remember to protect your bed sheets). Rinse the treatment out thoroughly and condition your hair as normal. Repeat 2-3 times per week for the best results. Each of the following recipes carries out 1 treatment.

Blend 1
2 tablespoons jojoba oil
10 drops of cypress
5 drops of lemon
5 drops of lavender
5 drops of rosemary

Blend 2
2 tablespoons grapeseed oil
5 drops of peppermint
5 drops of lavender
5 drops of cypress
5 drops of juniper berry
5 drops of lemon

Blend 3
2 tablespoons coconut oil
10 drops of lemon
10 drops of lavender
5 drops of peppermint

Blend 4
2 tablespoons sweet almond oil
10 drops of cypress
10 drops of rosemary
5 drops of grapefruit

❧ Treatment Shampoo ❧

Blend all ingredients together in a bowl and mix thoroughly. Apply to wet hair and massage into the scalp and hair. You may need to include more base shampoo depending on the length and thickness of your hair. The following formulas are for 1 treatment on medium length hair.

Blend 1
1 tablespoon unscented natural shampoo
1 teaspoon apple cider vinegar
6 drops of lemon
4 drops of cypress

Blend 2
1 tablespoon unscented natural shampoo
1 tablespoon coconut milk
4 drops of rosemary
4 drops of peppermint
2 drops of juniper berry

❧ Treatment Masks ❧

Adding a mask treatment to your healthy hair regime can really boost results by helping to further condition, nourish and improve the texture of hair. Blend all ingredients in a small bowl and mix thoroughly. Apply to damp, clean hair. Divide the hair into section and massage the mask into the hair and scalp, paying particular attention to the ends. Leave on for 1 hour and thoroughly rinse and condition hair as normal. Repeat twice per week. Each of the following recipes is for 1 treatment on medium length hair.

Blend 1
1 tablespoon raw unprocessed honey
Juice from ½ lemon
1 teaspoon jojoba oil
10 drops of rosemary
4 drops of lavender

Blend 2
1 tablespoon baking soda
1 tablespoon apple cider vinegar
5 drops of lemon
5 drops of peppermint
5 drops of cypress

Hands & Nails

The skin on our hands is actually the first tell tale sign of ageing skin, and because our hands do so much for us each day, it is vitally important to take good care of them. The prolonged use of harsh detergents, soaps, chemical-laden cosmetics and extreme winter elements can have a devastating effect on the hands, so keeping them protected with natural ingredients should be part of your regular beauty regime.

Our nails are just as delicate and therefore can be weakened by immersing the hands in soapy water, using harsh nail polish remover, prolonged use of household cleaning products and cold winters. Thankfully, essential oils not only help strengthen and thicken weak nails, but they can also condition and nourish our hands returning them to a healthy condition.

Essential oils for hands & nails; Benzoin, Cypress, Eucalyptus, Frankincense, Geranium, Lavender, Lemon, Lemongrass, Marjoram, Myrrh, Neroli, Patchouli, Peppermint, Rose, Sandalwood, Thyme.

Carrier oils for hands & nails; Sweet Almond, Apricot Kernel, Borage Seed, Coconut, Evening Primrose, Jojoba, Macadamia, Rosehip.

❧ Massage Oils ❧

Blend all ingredients together and mix thoroughly. Pour into the palm of the hand and gently rub both hands together to evenly spread the formula. Massage into the hands and fingers using small, circular movements. Leave to absorb into the skin, do not wash off. Repeat daily.

Mature Hands Blend 1
2 tablespoons coconut oil
4 drops of myrrh
4 drops of frankincense
4 drops of rose
4 drops of sandalwood

Mature Hands Blend 2
2 tablespoons sweet almond oil
4 drops of rosewood
4 drops of jasmine
4 drops of lavender
4 drops of frankincense

Soften & Nourish Hands Blend 1

2 tablespoons jojoba oil
4 drops of patchouli
4 drops of geranium
4 drops of lavender
4 drops of benzoin

Soften & Nourish Hands Blend 2

2 tablespoons sweet almond oil
2 vitamin E capsules
4 drops of lemon
4 drops of sandalwood
4 drops of peppermint
4 drops of myrrh

Aches & Pains Hand Blend 1

2 tablespoons jojoba oil
4 drops of chamomile
4 drops of marjoram
4 drops of eucalyptus
4 drops of juniper

Aches & Pains Hand Blend 2

2 tablespoons coconut oil
4 drops of lemongrass
4 drops of peppermint
4 drops of rosemary
4 drops of thyme

Hand Rejuvenator Blend 1

2 tablespoons sweet almond oil
4 drops of grapefruit
4 drops of geranium
4 drops of rosemary
4 drops of lavender

Hand Rejuvenator Blend 2

2 tablespoons macadamia
4 drops of peppermint
4 drops of cypress
4 drops of lemon
4 drops of neroli

Overnight Blend 1

2 tablespoons extra virgin olive oil
4 drops of jojoba oil
4 drops of geranium
4 drops of rose
4 drops of bergamot
4 drops of chamomile

Overnight Blend 2

2 tablespoons evening primrose
2 vitamin E capsules
4 drops of lavender
4 drops of eucalyptus
4 drops of geranium
4 drops of frankincense

Strengthen/Thicken Nails Blend 1

1 teaspoon jojoba oil
4 drops of lavender

Strengthen/Thicken Nails Blend 2

1 teaspoon olive oil
2 drops of lemon
2 drops of myrrh

Nourish/Condition Nails Blend 1

1 teaspoon extra virgin olive oil
2 drops of lavender
2 drops of lavender
2 drops of lemon

Dry Cuticles Blend

1 teaspoon rosehip oil
4 drops of lavender

Nourish/Condition Nails Blend 2

½ teaspoon jojoba oil
1 vitamin E capsule
3 drops of frankincense
1 drop of lavender

Nail Infection Around Nail

1 teaspoon coconut oil
2 drops of tea tree

❧ Hand Scrubs ❧

Blend all ingredients together in a small bowl and mix thoroughly. Massage into hands, applying gentle circular movements around the outside of the hands and fingers, the palms, in between the fingers and around each nail. Wash off in warm water, dry thoroughly and follow with a massage oil or a hand cream. Repeat 2-3 times per week.

Blend 1

1 tablespoon extra virgin olive oil
Juice from 1 lemon
½ tablespoon brown sugar
4 drops of grapefruit
4 drops of peppermint
2 drops of neroli
2 drops of lavender

Blend 2

2 vitamin E capsules
1 tablespoon jojoba oil
Juice from ½ lemon
4 drops of frankincense
4 drops of myrrh
2 drops of lemon
2 drops of rosemary

❧ Hand Masks ❧

Blend all ingredients together in a small bowl and mix thoroughly. Apply over the wrist, hands and fingers. Leave for 10 minutes and rinse off in warm water, follow with a massage oil or hand cream.

Blend 1
1 tablespoon raw honey
1 teaspoon rosehip oil
5 drops of lemon
5 drops of rosemary
5 drops of geranium

Blend 2
½ ripe avocado (mashed)
1 tablespoon raw honey
1 tablespoon extra virgin olive oil
5 drops of sandalwood
5 drops of myrrh
5 drops of frankincense

❧ Hand Soak ❧

A hand soak in warm water can be particularly useful for individuals suffering from tired, aching hands. At the end of the day, fill a large bowl of warm to hot water, add the essential oils and soak for 20 minutes.

Blend 1
1 tablespoon sweet almond oil
5 drops of peppermint
3 drops of marjoram
3 drops of lavender
1 drop of lemon

Blend 2
1 tablespoon evening primrose oil
5 drops of ylang ylang
4 drops of geranium
3 drops of chamomile

Blend 3
1 tablespoon jojoba oil
10 drops of chamomile
2 drops of lavender

Blend 4
1 tablespoon extra virgin olive oil
5 drops of marjoram
5 drops of bergamot
2 drops of lemon

❧ Hand Creams ❧

Blend all ingredients together and mix thoroughly (some ingredients may need to be melted and returned to solid form, depending on recipe). Apply to hands daily or whenever they feel dry. Always ensure to protect hands in winter elements. Each recipe should last approximately 5-6 days, store in a cool, dry place.

Mature Skin Blend

1 tablespoon solid raw virgin coconut oil
1 tablespoon rosehip oil
10 drops of frankincense
2 drops of myrrh
2 drops of sandalwood
melt the coconut oil first, add the remaining oils and allow to solidify in a cool place for 12 hours.

Soften & Nourish Blend

1 tablespoon solid shea butter
2 vitamin E capsules
8 drops of lavender
6 drops of geranium
melt the shea butter first, add the remaining oils and allow to solidify in a cool place for 12 hours.

Rejuvenate Hand Blend

1 tablespoon beeswax pellets
1 teaspoon solid raw virgin coconut oil
10 drops of peppermint
4 drops of lemongrass
melt the coconut oil and beeswax first, add the remaining oils and allow to solidify in a cool place for 12 hours.

Aches & Pains Blend

1 tablespoon solid shea butter
1 tablespoon jojoba oil
8 drops of marjoram
2 drops of lavender
2 drops of rosemary
2 drops of eucalyptus
melt the shea butter first, add the remaining oils and allow to solidify in a cool place for 12 hours.

Overnight Blend

1 tablespoon beeswax pellets

1 tablespoon solid raw virgin coconut oil

1 teaspoon rosehip oil

6 drops of bergamot

4 drops of geranium

4 drops of frankincense

melt the beeswax and coconut oil first, add the remaining oils and allow to solidify in a cool place for 12 hours.

Oily Skin

Oily or congested skin is a condition that occurs due to over-reactive sebaceous glands. It has the following characteristics;

♦ Enlarged pores
♦ Dull and sallow skin color
♦ Shiny appearance
♦ Blemishes and blackheads are common

When choosing essential oils for oily skin, choose oils that help to control excess facial oil, balance the skin's oil production, have astringent properties to close and tighten pores and help to treat blemishes.

Essential oils for oily skin include; Bergamot, Cedarwood, Clary Sage, Frankincense, Geranium, Grapefruit, Juniper, Lavender, Lemon, Lemongrass, Mandarin, Orange (Sweet), Petitgrain, Rosemary, Tea Tree, Ylang Ylang.

Carrier oils for oily skin include; Apricot Kernel, Coconut, Grapeseed, Hazelnut, Jojoba.

❧ Facial Oils ❧

Blend all the ingredients together and mix thoroughly. Apply the formula to a cleansed face and neck, and gently massage using small circular movements. Leave the oils to absorb into the skin cells, do not wash off. Carry out the treatment twice per day, once in the morning and again at night. At night, a facial oil can be substituted with a facial moisturizer (recipes below) if you prefer. The following recipes will yield enough for 1 treatment. Where coconut oil is used in these recipes, make sure to use Raw Virgin Coconut Oil as it is the best form of coconut oil to use for the skin. Melt it by placing an even tablespoon into a cup, place the cup into a saucepan of boiling water, and continue to boil the water on the heat until the coconut oil has melted. Never melt in the microwave.

Blend 1
1 tablespoon coconut oil
8 drops of cypress oil
3 drops of lemon
3 drops of cedarwood

Blend 2
1 tablespoon coconut oil
8 drops of ylang ylang
8 drops of juniper

Blend 3

1 tablespoon hazelnut oil
4 drops of bergamot
4 drops of petitgrain
4 drops of cypress
2 drops of rosemary

Blend 4

1 tablespoon jojoba oil
6 drops of orange
6 drops of lemon
4 drops of geranium

❧ Facial Cleansers ❧

Blend all ingredients together and mix thoroughly. Apply the formula to the face and neck, and massage into the skin using outward circular movements. Leave to absorb into the skin for 2 minutes. Gently remove all traces of oil preferably using a wet muslin cloth soaked in warm water. A small, soft face towel can be used as an alternative. Repeat twice per day, once in the morning and again at night before applying a facial oil or moisturizer. The following recipes will yield enough for 1 treatment. Regarding coconut oil, please refer to 'Facial Oils' above for instructions on how to prepare.

Blend 1

2 tablespoons of aloe vera gel
1 teaspoon hazelnut oil
4 drops of lavender
3 drops of petitgrain
2 drops of juniper
2 drops of ylang ylang

Blend 2

1 tablespoon of plain yogurt
2 teaspoons of lemon juice
2 drops of clary sage
2 drops of mandarin
2 drops of rosemary

Blend 3

20ml coconut oil
2 drops of tea tree
2 drops of bergamot
2 drops of geranium
2 drops of lemongrass

Blend 4

1 tablespoon aloe vera gel
1 tablespoon veg glycerin
2 tablespoons witch hazel
2 drops of tea tree
2 drops of rosemary
2 drops of petitgrain
1 drop of lemongrass

❧ Facial Toners ❧

Blend all ingredients in a glass bottle and shake well to combine. You can use a spray bottle if you wish but it is not necessary. Always add the hydrosol (flower water) first and then follow with the essential oils. Distilled water is a great alternative to hydrosols but always ensure you use distilled water (tap water may contain chemicals or bacteria). If you are using a spray bottle, hold it 3 to 4 inches away from the face, close your eyes and spray. Do not wipe off. If you are using a normal bottle, soak a cotton pad with the toner and gently pat all over the face and neck. Apply each time after cleansing, exfoliating or a face mask. The following recipes will yield enough for approximately 2 to 3 days.

Blend 1
1 cup witch hazel
10 drops of lavender
10 drops of juniper

Blend 2
½ cup witch hazel
½ cup distilled water
4 drops of tea tree
4 drops of lemongrass
2 drops of petitgrain
2 drops of rosemary

Blend 3
1 cup distilled water
2 tablespoons aloe vera juice
5 drops of ylang ylang
5 drops of juniper
5 drops of orange (sweet)

Blend 4
2 tablespoons apple cider vinegar
½ cup distilled water
8 drops of cypress
4 drops of clary sage
2 drops of grapefruit
2 drops of bergamot

❧ Facial Moisturizers ❧

Blend all ingredients together and mix thoroughly. After cleansing and toning, apply the formula onto the face and neck, and massage into the skin, using small, gentle circular movements with the fingertips. If you are applying a day blend, allow the oils to absorb into the skin for 2 minutes before applying makeup. Repeat twice per day, once in the morning and again at night. A moisturizer may be substituted for a facial oil (recipes above) if you wish. The following recipes will yield enough for 1 – 2 treatments. Regarding coconut oil, please refer to 'Facial Oils' above for instructions on how to prepare.

Day Blend 1

1 tablespoon jojoba oil
1 teaspoon witch hazel
5 drops of tea tree
5 drops of lemongrass

Day Blend 2

1 tablespoon coconut oil
5 drops of bergamot
2 drops of grapefruit
2 drops of cypress

Night Blend 1

1 tablespoon apricot kernel oil
8 drops of petitgrain
6 drops of lemon
4 drops of juniper
2 drops of frankincense
2 drops of clary sage

Night Blend 2

1 tablespoon coconut oil
10ml tamanu oil
10 drops of rosemary
6 drops of lemongrass

❧ Facial Scrubs ❧

Combine all ingredients in a small bowl, mix thoroughly and use immediately. Massage the blend gently into the skin as you would the facial cleanser. Leave on the skin for 2 minutes and wash off with warm water. Carry out this treatment once per week. The following recipes will yield enough for 1 treatment. Regarding coconut oil, please refer to 'Facial Oils' above for instructions on how to prepare.

Blend 1

1 tablespoon baking soda
1 teaspoon fresh lemon juice
1 teaspoon jojoba oil
10 drops of lemon
10 drops of geranium

Blend 2

1 tablespoon brown sugar
1 teaspoon hazelnut oil
4 drops of mandarin
4 drops of juniper
4 drops of lavender
2 drops of tea tree

Blend 3

2 tablespoons ground oats
1 tablespoon extra virgin olive oil
8 drops of orange
4 drops of bergamot
4 drops of lemon

Blend 4

1 tablespoon manuka honey
1 teaspoon granulated sugar
8 drops of ylang ylang
8 drops of juniper
6 drops of lavender

❧ Facial Masks ❧

Blend all ingredients in a small bowl, mix thoroughly and use immediately. Apply the formula with either a mask brush or clean fingers, after the skin has been cleansed. Leave on for 15 to 20 minutes and wash off with warm water. Pat dry the face, follow with a toner and moisturizer or facial oil. Apply a face mask once every week. The following recipes will yield enough for 1 treatment.

Blend 1
1 small banana mashed up
1 tablespoon manuka honey
1 teaspoon lemon juice
5 drops of juniper
5 drops of petitgrain

Blend 2
2 egg whites
1 tablespoon lemon juice
5 drops of frankincense
5 drops of bergamot

Blend 3
2 tablespoons plain organic yogurt
10 drops of petitgrain
10 drops of lemon
10 drops of orange

Blend 4
30ml coconut oil
1 tablespoon manuka honey
1 tablespoon baking soda
6 drops of tea tree
6 drops of bergamot
6 drops of geranium
3 drops of lemon

❧ Facial Sauna ❧

Fill a large bowl with boiling water, add the chosen essential oils, place a towel around your head and lean towards the water (closing off the sides with the towel). The steam can burn your skin so hold your head as close as is comfortable. Close eyes and inhale deeply for 7 – 10 minutes.

Blend 1
1 large bowl of boiling water
2 drops of cypress
2 drops of lemon
2 drops of juniper
1 drop of bergamot

Blend 2
1 large bowl of boiling water
3 drops of tea tree
3 drops of lavender

Blend 3

1 large bowl of boiling water
2 drops of lemongrass
2 drops of grapefruit
1 drop of lemon
1 drop of bergamot

Blend 4

1 large bowl of boiling water
3 drops of geranium
3 drops of rosemary

Stretch Marks

Stretch marks are small tears in the deep layers of the skin that usually occur as a result of pregnancy or rapid fluctuations in weight. Common areas for stretch marks are the abdomen, hips, buttocks and breasts. There are several essential oils that you can use, particularly ones that have healing and tissue regenerating properties.

Essential oils for stretch marks; Frankincense, Jasmine, Lavender, Mandarin, Myrrh, Neroli, Patchouli, Rose.

Carrier oils for stretch marks; Sweet Almond, Borage Seed, Carrot, Coconut, Evening Primrose, Jojoba, Rosehip Seed, Wheatgerm.

❧ Massage Oils ❧

Blend all ingredients together and mix thoroughly. Apply the formula to the area in question and rub into the skin in circular movements. Allow the blend to absorb into the skin, do not wash off. Repeat twice each day, once in the morning and again in the evening. The following recipes will make treatments for 1 day.

Blend 1
1 tablespoon melted raw virgin coconut oil
1 tablespoon rosehip oil
1 vitamin E capsule
8 drops of neroli
8 drops of myrrh
4 drops of lavender

Blend 2
1 tablespoon sweet almond oil
1 tablespoon wheatgerm oil
5 drops of carrot oil
1 teaspoon jojoba oil
8 drops of lavender
8 drops of mandarin

Blend 3
1 tablespoon jojoba oil
1 tablespoon evening primrose oil
6 drops of frankincense
6 drops of myrrh
4 drops of rose
2 drops of neroli
2 drops of lavender

Blend 4
1 tablespoon wheatgerm oil
1 teaspoon coconut oil
1 teaspoon rosehip oil
1 teaspoon jojoba oil
5 drops of mandarin
5 drops of jasmine

11
Aromatherapy for Health

Arthritis

A disorder of the skeletal system, arthritis is the inflammation of one or more joints and can be a very painful and crippling condition. Symptoms include swelling, stiffness and/or inflammation, and joints commonly affected are the wrists, knees and hips. Essential oils that provide natural pain relief and contain anti-inflammatory properties are an effective and beneficial treatment for the symptoms of arthritis.

Essential oils for arthritis; Basil, Cedarwood, Chamomile (Roman), Cypress, Eucalyptus, Geranium, Ginger, Juniper, Lavender, Lemon, Lemongrass, Marjoram, Peppermint, Rosemary.

Carrier oils for arthritis; Sweet Almond, Avocado, Coconut, Grapeseed.

❧ Massage Oils ❧

Blend all ingredients together and mix thoroughly. Massage the whole body paying particular attention to the affected limb. Repeat in the morning and again at night. Leave the oils to absorb into the skin, do not wash off. The following recipes will yield enough for 1 treatment.

Pain Relief Blend 1
3 tablespoons grapeseed oil
8 drops of marjoram
5 drops of rosemary
2 drops of eucalyptus

Pain Relief Blend 2
3 tablespoons melted coconut oil
6 drops of chamomile
6 drops of eucalyptus
3 drops of ginger

Inflammation Blend 1

3 tablespoons sweet almond oil
5 drops of cypress
5 drops of peppermint
5 drops of lemon

General Arthritis Blend 1

3 tablespoons grapeseed oil
6 drops of grapefruit
4 drops of cypress
5 drops of chamomile

Inflammation Blend 2

3 tablespoons grapeseed oil
5 drops of lavender
5 drops of rosemary

General Arthritis Blend 2

3 tablespoons avocado oil
5 drops of frankincense
5 drops of cedarwood
5 drops of lemon

❧ Bath Oils ❧

Blend all ingredients together and mix thoroughly. Add the Epsom salts first and fill the bath. Once filled, add the essential oils, agitate the water to disperse the oils around the bath, and soak for 20 minutes. The following recipes will yield enough for 1 treatment.

Joint Pain Relief Blend 1

1 cup Epsom salts
1 tablespoon grapeseed oil
4 drops of juniper
4 drops of cypress
2 drops of rosemary

Joint Pain Relief Blend 2

1 cup Epsom salts
1 tablespoon sweet almond oil
6 drops of peppermint
4 drops of marjoram

Inflammation Blend 1

1 cup Epsom salts
1 tablespoon olive oil
8 drops of lemongrass
2 drops of peppermint

Inflammation Blend 2

1 cup Epsom salts
1 tablespoon grapeseed oil
4 drops of chamomile
4 drops of marjoram
2 drops of rosemary

❧ Cold Compress ❧

Prepare a bowl of cold water, add your chosen essential oils and place the compress into the water to soak for 2 minutes. Remove and wring out any excess water. Apply over the affected area for 1 to 2 hours or until it has warmed to body heat, at which time it can be replaced with a fresh one.

Pain Relief Blend
10 drops of marjoram
3 drops of rosemary
2 drops of eucalyptus

Inflammation Blend
10 drops of peppermint
5 drops of chamomile

Athlete's Foot

Athlete's foot is a common fungal infection of the foot, characterized by red, itchy, scaly skin. It usually begins between the toes and sometimes spreads to other parts of the feet. Essential oils with anti-fungal and anti-inflammatory properties are the most effective in treating this contagious skin disorder.

Essential oils for athlete's foot; Cedarwood, Geranium, Lavender. Lemon, Myrrh, Peppermint, Tea Tree.

Carrier oils for athlete's foot; Sweet Almond, Avocado, Coconut, Grapeseed, Olive.

❧ Massage Oils ❧

Blend all ingredients together and mix thoroughly. Massage the formula into cleansed feet, making sure to massage in between each toe. Thoroughly wash hands after use. Leave the oils to absorb into the skin, do not wash off. Repeat each night before bedtime. The following recipes will yield enough for 1 treatment.

Blend 1
1 tablespoon melted coconut oil (raw virgin)
10 drops of tea tree

Blend 2
1 tablespoon extra virgin olive oil
4 drops of geranium
4 drops of myrrh
2 drops of lavender

Blend 3
1 tablespoon grapeseed oil
6 drops of lemon
2 drops of geranium
2 drops of peppermint

Blend 4
1 tablespoon melted coconut oil
1 teaspoon apple cider vinegar
8 drops of tea tree
2 drops of peppermint

Bites & Stings

Bites & stings can cause painful reactions and feelings of irritation and discomfort. Essential oils that have anti-inflammatory, antiseptic and pain relieving properties are the most effective ones to use as they help to reduce inflammation, ease the sting, clean the wound and speed up the healing process.

Essential oils for bites and stings; Basil, Chamomile (Roman), Eucalyptus, Lavender, Peppermint, Rosemary, Tea Tree, Thyme.

Carrier oils for bites and stings; Aloe Vera (not a carrier oil but a very effective treatment nonetheless), Borage Seed, Coconut.

❧ Insect Stings ❧

Very gently remove the sting if it is visible. Apply the blend every 1-2 hours until symptoms begin to ease.

Blend 1
1 drop of neat lavender directly over the area

Blend 2
1 teaspoon aloe vera gel
1 drop of chamomile
1 drop of lavender

❧ Bee Stings ❧

Very gently remove the sting if it is visible. Clean the wound with cool water and apply one of the blends below. Repeat 3 times per day for 2-3 days.

Blend 1
1 drop of neat chamomile directly over the sting

Blend 2

1 teaspoon baking soda

½ teaspoon apply cider vinegar

2 drops of lavender

leave on for 30 minutes and wash off with cool water

Blend 3

1 teaspoon aloe vera gel

2 drops of lavender

1 drop of chamomile

Blend 4

1 teaspoon aloe vera gel

1 drop of peppermint

1 drop of lavender

1 drop of chamomile

❧ Mosquito Bites ❧

Apply the blend every 2-3 hours for 2 days or until symptoms subside.

Blend 1

1 drop of neat lavender oil directly over the bite

Blend 2

1 teaspoon aloe vera gel

4 drops of chamomile

Blend 3

1 teaspoon apple cider vinegar

2 drops of thyme

2 drops of lavender

Blend 4

1 teaspoon fresh lemon juice

1 drop of basil

1 drop of peppermint

1 drop of tea tree

1 drop of lavender

❧ Compress for Bites & Stings ❧

Fill a bowl of cold water followed by essential oils and immerse a compress. Soak for 5 minutes to allow the oils to absorb into the compress. Ring out any excess water and apply directly over the bite or sting for 20 minutes. If you need to re-immerse the compress in the water to cool it down you can do so.

Blend 1
10 drops of chamomile

Blend 2
5 drops of chamomile
5 drops of lavender

Blend 3
5 drops of lavender
5 drops of peppermint

Blend 4
5 drops of thyme
5 drops of basil

Blisters

Blisters can appear on the skin for a variety of reasons; burns, badly fitted shoes, friction from repeated use of metal tools, sunburn etc. Not only are they a painful skin condition but they are prone to infection if not properly looked after. Essential oils that have both antibacterial and analgesic properties are the most effective.

Essential oils for blisters; Chamomile (Roman), Lavender, Tea Tree.

Carrier oils for blisters; Coconut, Evening Primrose, Olive.

❧ Massage Oils ❧

Blend all ingredients using a 50:50 dilution (one part essential oil to one part carrier oil). Pat the formula gently onto the blister, making sure not to burst it. If the blister has already burst, the formula can be applied in the same way. Repeat the treatment several times per day until the blister has cleared. The following recipes will yield enough for 1 treatment.

Blend 1
½ teaspoon melted coconut oil
1 drop of lavender
1 drop of tea tree
1 drop of chamomile

Blend 2
½ teaspoon extra virgin olive oil
3 drops of lavender

Blend 3
½ teaspoon melted coconut oil
2 drops of chamomile
1 drop of tea tree

Blend 4
½ teaspoon extra virgin olive oil
2 drops of tea tree
1 drop of lavender

Cold Sores

Cold sores, also known as herpes simplex, are caused by the herpes virus that can lie dormant in the nerve cells for long periods of time between breakouts. The virus can become reactivated for a number of different reasons including stress, both emotional and physical, too much sun exposure, poor diet, depression and more. The first sign of a cold sore would be a tingling sensation or itch, a red bump will then appear, closely followed by the formation of a blister. Cold sores can be painful and itchy, and can be a cause of embarrassment for sufferers. Essential oils have proven to be an effective treatment but must always be diluted in a carrier oil and never ingested.

Essential oils for cold sores; Geranium, Lavender, Lemon, Tea Tree.

Carrier oils for cold sores; Coconut, Evening Primrose, Olive.

❧ Cotton Bud ❧

Blend ingredients together in a tightly sealed dark bottle. Wet a cotton bud with warm water and place one drop of the mixture onto the cotton bud. Dab the cold sore directly. Never place the cotton bud back into the bottle containing the essential oil blend. Reapply several times per day until the cold sore has cleared up. The following recipes will yield enough for 1 treatment.

Blend 1
1 teaspoon olive oil
5 drops of tea tree

Blend 2
1 teaspoon fractionated coconut oil
5 drops of geranium

Coughs

A cough occurs when an individual has a respiratory tract infection caused by a virus. It can accompany a common cold, the flu, hay fever, laryngitis, or in more severe cases, pneumonia or asthma. Coughs are usually short term but can be the sign of an underlying health problem if it persists for longer than 6 to 8 weeks, at which time a doctor should be consulted. Essential oils that have expectorant properties are ideal to use as they help to clear mucus along the respiratory tract.

Essential oils for coughs; Bergamot, Black Pepper, Cedarwood, Eucalyptus, Frankincense, Lavender, Lemon, Lemongrass, Myrrh, Peppermint, Pine, Rosemary, Sandalwood, Tea Tree, Thyme.

Carrier oils for coughs; Coconut, Grapeseed, Olive, Sunflower.

❧ Massage Oils ❧

Blend all ingredients together and mix thoroughly. Massage the formula into the throat, chest and back of the neck. Leave the oils to absorb into the skin, do not wash off. Carry out the treatment every day until the cough subsides. The following recipes will yield enough for 1 treatment.

Blend 1
1 tablespoon olive oil
6 drops of lavender
6 drops of eucalyptus

Blend 2
1 tablespoon grapeseed oil
5 drops of peppermint
4 drops of lemongrass
3 drops of black pepper

Blend 3
1 tablespoon coconut oil
5 drops of eucalyptus
5 drops of peppermint
2 drops of thyme

Blend 4
1 tablespoon olive oil
5 drops of bergamot
4 drops of lavender
3 drops of eucalyptus

❧ Diffuser/Oil Burner ❧

Place the water and essential oils at the top of the diffuser and light the candle below. Allow 10 to 15 minutes for the aroma to fill the room. Sit back and take several deep breaths for approximately 10 minutes. The following blends should only be used during the day due to their stimulating properties.

Blend 1
4 drops of eucalyptus
2 drops of peppermint

Blend 2
3 drops of bergamot
2 drops of lavender
1 drop of thyme

❧ Inhalations ❧

Prepare a bowl of steaming hot water, add your chosen essential oils, cover your head with a towel, close your eyes and inhale the aroma of the oils for 2 to 3 minutes. Repeat once per day until symptoms subside.

Blend 1
4 drops of eucalyptus
2 drops of bergamot

Blend 2
3 drops of peppermint
2 drops of myrrh
1 drop of thyme

❧ Bath Oils ❧

Blend all ingredients together and add to the water once the bath has been filled. Agitate the water to disperse the oils, and soak for 20 minutes. Because of the stimulating properties in some of the oils used, it is best to use these recipes in the morning or during the day.

Blend 1
1 tablespoon olive oil
8 drops of myrrh
4 drops of eucalyptus

Blend 2
1 tablespoon grapeseed oil
6 drops of bergamot
4 drops of peppermint
2 drops of lavender

Cystitis

Cystitis is inflammation of the membrane lining of the urinary bladder, and is more common in women than in men, due to women having shorter urethras. The symptoms of cystitis include pain in the lower part of the abdomen, a desire to pass urine frequently, pain on urination, and the passage of cloudy or foul smelling urine. Appropriate essential oils can be used to gently massage over the lower abdomen, on hot compresses, and in external washes and baths.

Essential oils for cystitis; Basil, Bergamot, Cedarwood, Chamomile (Roman), Cypress, Eucalyptus, Fennel, Juniper, Lavender, Rosemary, Sandalwood, Tea Tree, Thyme.

Carrier oils for cystitis; Sweet Almond, Coconut, Grapeseed.

❧ Massage Oils ❧

Blend all ingredients together and mix thoroughly. Gently massage the formula into the lower abdomen, lower back and hips using circular, clockwise movements. Repeat once in the morning and once at night until symptoms subside. Leave the oils to absorb into the skin, do not wash off. The following recipes will yield enough for 1 treatment.

Blend 1
1 tablespoon grapeseed oil
4 drops of sandalwood
4 drops of lavender
2 drops of chamomile

Blend 2
1 tablespoon coconut oil
3 drops of cypress
3 drops of thyme
3 drops of cedarwood
1 drop of basil

Blend 3
1 tablespoon sweet almond oil
4 drops of rosemary
2 drops of fennel
2 drops of lavender
2 drops of cypress

Blend 4
1 tablespoon grapeseed oil
4 drops of chamomile
3 drops of bergamot
2 drops of juniper
1 drop of tea tree

❧ Sitz Bath ❧

Blend and mix ingredients thoroughly. Fill the bath water (tepid water only) up the waist, add the essential oils, agitate the water to disperse the oils and sit in the bath for approximately 20 minutes.

Blend 1
1 tablespoon evening primrose oil
4 drops of rosemary
4 drops of bergamot

Blend 2
1 tablespoon grapeseed oil
3 drops of lavender
3 drops of cypress
2 drops of eucalyptus

Blend 3
1 tablespoon melted olive oil
4 drops of juniper
2 drops of bergamot
2 drops of tea tree

Blend 4
1 tablespoon sweet almond oil
5 drops of lavender
2 drops of rosemary
1 drop of cypress

❧ Hot Compress ❧

Prepare a bowl of hot water and add your chosen essential oils. Place the compress into the water and allow to soak for 2 minutes. Remove and wring out any excess water. Apply over the lower abdomen or lower back (both is also possible) and leave for 1 to 2 hours, or until it has warmed to body heat, at which time it can be replaced with a fresh one.

Blend 1
6 drops of bergamot
3 drops of rosemary
1 drop of lavender

Blend 2
5 drops of juniper
4 drops of cypress
1 drop of eucalyptus

Depression

While essential oils are not known to cure depression, they can certainly be an effective way to relieve some of the symptoms in mild to moderate cases. Aromatherapy blends can help with mental fatigue, mood swings, restlessness, insomnia, and anxiety. Through inhalation, essential oils have a strong and immediate effect on the emotions, lifting and enhancing a person's mood or outlook.

Essential oils for depression; Basil, Bergamot, Cedarwood, Chamomile (Roman), Clary Sage, Cypress, Frankincense, Geranium, Grapefruit, Jasmine, Lavender, Lemon, Lemongrass, Marjoram, Melissa, Neroli, Orange (Sweet), Peppermint, Petitgrain, Rose, Rosemary, Sandalwood, Ylang Ylang.

Carrier Oils for depression; Sweet Almond, Apricot Kernel, Avocado, Coconut, Evening Primrose, Grapeseed, Jojoba, Olive, Peach Kernel, Wheatgerm.

❧ Massage Oils ❧

Blend all ingredients together and mix thoroughly. Massage into the body as and when is needed. A carrier oil of your choice can be substituted for any of the ones below. The following recipes will yield enough for 1 treatment. Repeat each morning.

Uplifting Blend 1
3 tablespoons sweet almond oil
5 drops of clary sage
5 drops of ylang ylang
5 drops of geranium
5 drops of sandalwood

Uplifting Blend 2
3 tablespoons jojoba oil
8 drops of bergamot
8 drops of lavender
2 drops of clary sage
2 drops of orange (sweet)

Calming Blend 1
3 tablespoons evening primrose oil
8 drops of cypress
6 drops of marjoram
4 drops of melissa

Calming Blend 2
3 tablespoons apricot kernel
8 drops of chamomile
6 drops of clary sage
6 drops of jasmine

Reduce Anxiety Blend 1

3 tablespoons coconut oil

10 drops of lavender

4 drops of bergamot

4 drops of clary sage

Reduce Anxiety Blend 2

3 tablespoons wheatgerm oil

8 drops of frankincense

2 drops of marjoram

2 drops of lavender

2 drops of chamomile

2 drops of ylang ylang

Mental Re-energizer Blend 1

3 tablespoons sweet almond oil

10 drops of basil

4 drops of peppermint

2 drops of rosemary

2 drops of cedarwood

Mental Re-energizer Blend 2

3 tablespoons coconut oil

6 drops of bergamot

6 drops of cypress

6 drops of peppermint

❧ Bath Oils ❧

Blend all ingredients together and mix thoroughly. Add to the bath after it has been filled. Agitate the water to disperse the oils. Soak for 20 minutes. Repeat as and when is needed. A carrier oil of your choice can be substituted for any of the ones below.

Uplifting Blend 1

1 tablespoon sweet almond oil

4 drops of bergamot

4 drops of orange (sweet)

4 drops of clary sage

2 drops of lemon

Uplifting Blend 2

1 tablespoon olive oil

5 drops of sandalwood

5 drops of orange (sweet)

2 drops of lemongrass

2 drops of cypress

Calming Blend 1

1 tablespoon grapeseed oil

10 drops of chamomile

4 drops of geranium

Calming Blend 2

1 tablespoon coconut oil

4 drops of basil

4 drops of lavender

4 drops of cedarwood

2 drops of melissa

Anxiety Reliever Blend 1
1 tablespoon sweet almond oil
6 drops of clary sage
6 drops of frankincense
2 drops of sandalwood
2 drops of lavender

Anxiety Reliever 2
1 tablespoon peach kernel oil
8 drops of ylang ylang
4 drops of jasmine
2 drops of geranium
1 drop of neroli

Mental Re-energizer Blend 1
1 tablespoon avocado oil
6 drops of lemon
6 drops of rosemary
6 drops of basil

Mental Re-energizer Blend 2
1 tablespoon grapeseed oil
4 drops of rosemary
4 drops of peppermint
4 drops of clary sage
4 drops of basil

❧ Treatment Spritz ❧

Blend all ingredients together in a spray body and mix thoroughly. Spray throughout the day whenever you feel the need. Always hold the bottle about 3 – 4 inches away from the face and close your eyes before spraying. The following recipes will yield enough for approximately 2 days. Shake well before use.

Uplifting Spritz
50ml distilled water
10 drops of grapefruit
4 drops of bergamot
4 drops of lemon
2 drops of rosemary

Calming Spritz
50ml distilled water
6 drops of lavender
6 drops of jasmine
6 drops of sandalwood
2 drops of ylang ylang

Anxiety Reliever Spritz
50ml distilled water
10 drops of lavender
4 drops of petitgrain
4 drops of geranium
2 drops of basil

Mental Re-energizer Spritz
50ml distilled water
10 drops of peppermint
10 drops of basil

❧ Diffuser/Oil Burner ❧

Fill the bowl at the top of the vaporizer with water, followed by your chosen essential oils. Light a small candle, and place it underneath. Allow the beautiful aroma to fill the room. Repeat as and when is needed.

Uplifting Blend
3 drops of ylang ylang
3 drops of bergamot
3 drops of orange (sweet)

Anxiety Reliever Blend
3 drops of marjoram
3 drops of basil
3 drops of grapefruit

Calming Blend
3 drops of chamomile
3 drops of lavender
3 drops of geranium

Mental Re-energizer Blend
3 drops of peppermint
3 drops of lemongrass
3 drops of rosemary

Diarrhea

Disruptions to the normal passage of food through the small and large intestines give rise to diarrhea. Viruses and bacteria, irritant drugs, poisons, and allergic reactions are among the common causes. Most attacks of diarrhea will clear up within a day or 2 (acute diarrhea) but if it persists for longer than 2 days (prolonged diarrhea), the body will start to become dehydrated and it would be best to consult a doctor to ensure there is not serious disorder of the intestines. In any case of diarrhea, plenty of water should be consumed. A massage over the abdomen with certain essential oils can assist with this problem.

Essential oils for diarrhea; Basil, Chamomile (Roman), Cypress, Eucalyptus, Geranium, Lavender, Lemon, Neroli, Orange, Peppermint.

Carrier oils for diarrhea; Sweet Almond, Avocado, Coconut, Grapeseed.

❧ Massage Oils ❧

Blend all ingredients together and mix thoroughly. Massage the formula in a clockwise motion around the abdomen. Carry out this treatment as soon as the diarrhea starts, and continue to massage the abdomen once per day thereafter, until the symptoms ease. The following recipes will yield enough for 1 treatment.

Blend 1
1 tablespoon grapeseed oil
4 drops of peppermint
3 drops of lavender
2 drops of chamomile
1 drop of eucalyptus

Blend 2
1 tablespoon sweet almond oil
5 drops of peppermint
5 drops of chamomile

Blend 3
1 tablespoon grapeseed oil
3 drops of cypress
3 drops of geranium
2 drops of chamomile
2 drops of orange

Blend 4
1 tablespoon avocado oil
6 drops of lavender
2 drops of neroli
1 drop of eucalyptus
1 drop of peppermint

Ear Infections

An ear infection usually occurs when a viral or bacterial infection such as a cold or flu causes mucus to build up in the middle ear, which then becomes infected. It can be a very painful experience for some people which usually clears up after 3 to 5 days. Essential oils are a natural treatment for ear infections, and ones containing antiviral, antiseptic and antibacterial properties should be used. Please note that essential oils must never be dropped inside the ear itself.

Essential oils for ear infections; Eucalyptus, Lavender, Lemon, Rosemary, Tea Tree.

Carrier oils for ear infections; Coconut, Grapeseed, Olive.

❧ Massage Oils ❧

Blend all ingredients together and mix thoroughly. Gently massage the formula around the outside, front and back of the ear, and down along the lymph nodes at the side of the neck. Always ensure that none of the blend is dropped into the ear. It is recommended to massage both ears, not just one. Carry out this treatment 3 to 4 times per day, especially before bedtime.

Blend 1
1 tablespoon melted coconut oil
4 drops of lavender
2 drops of eucalyptus

Blend 2
1 tablespoon extra virgin olive oil
3 drops of rosemary
3 drops of tea tree

Eczema

Eczema is a non-infectious inflammatory disorder of the skin that takes the form of redness, blistering, crusting and scaling. It is a condition which is varied in the way it manifests. A well known type of eczema, which begins in infancy and childhood, is called topic eczema and tends to run in families where there is asthma, migraine or hay fever. Allergic eczema is usually due to food allergy, and occupational eczema is normally caused by skin irritants such as liquid detergents and soap powders.

Stress is involved in almost all cases of eczema, so it is important to use oils which help to combat stress as well as those which act by treating the skin directly. Many people with eczema find that carrier oils can sometimes make the condition worse, so for the purpose of these recipes I have only included coconut oil (raw virgin) as it is both nourishing and healing.

Essential oils for eczema; Bergamot, Chamomile (Roman), Frankincense, Geranium, Juniper, Lavender, Melissa, Neroli, Rose.

Carrier oils for eczema; Aloe Vera (not a carrier oil as such but it is still a very effective treatment for eczema), Coconut.

❧ Massage Oils ❧

Blend all ingredients together and mix thoroughly. Massage the formula into the affected area and leave the oils to absorb into the skin, do not wash off. Repeat twice a day, once in the morning and once in the evening. Depending on the area being treated, you may need to add more coconut oil or aloe vera gel. The recipes below will yield enough for 1 treatment on a small area. Because eczema is a sensitive skin disorder, less essential oils are used.

Blend 1
1 tablespoon melted coconut oil
2 drops of chamomile
2 drops of lavender
2 drops of neroli

Blend 2
1 tablespoon aloe vera gel
3 drops of chamomile
2 drops of frankincense
1 drop of geranium

Blend 3

1 tablespoon aloe vera gel

2 drops of melissa

2 drops of neroli

2 drops of juniper

Blend 4

1 tablespoon melted coconut oil

2 drops of bergamot

2 drops of rose

2 chamomile

❧ Cold Compress ❧

Prepare a bowl of cold water and add your chosen essential oils. Place the compress into the water and allow to soak for 2 minutes. Remove and wring out any excess water. Apply over the affected area and leave for 1 hour. Each time the compress starts to warm to body heat, dip it in the water to refresh and apply again.

Blend 1

2 drops of chamomile

2 drops of lavender

Blend 2

3 drops of chamomile

1 drop of bergamot

❧ Bath Oils ❧

Blend and mix the ingredients together. Fill the bath with lukewarm water (not hot). Once the bath has been filled, add the essential oils, agitate the water to disperse the oils, and soak for 20 minutes.

Blend 1

1 tablespoon melted coconut oil

6 drops of chamomile

4 drops of lavender

Blend 2

1 tablespoon melted coconut oil

3 drops of geranium

3 drops of bergamot

3 drops of frankincense

1 drop of lavender

Blend 3

1 tablespoon melted coconut oil

4 drops of neroli

3 drops of juniper

3 drops of lavender

Blend 4

1 tablespoon melted coconut oil

5 drops of melissa

2 drops of frankincense

2 drops of neroli

1 drop of bergamot

Exam Preparation

Certain essential oils are known to improve concentration levels and stimulate the brain, thus helping to focus the mind during study time.

Essential oils for exam preparation; Basil, Bergamot, Ginger, Grapefruit, Lavender, Lemon, Peppermint, Rosemary.

Carrier oils for exam preparation; Sweet Almond, Evening Primrose.

❧ Massage Oils ❧

Blend all ingredients together and mix thoroughly. Massage the formula into the back of the neck and shoulders. Do not wash off. The following recipes will make 1 treatment. Please note that stimulating oils such as rosemary and basil should be avoided in the evening time so as not to disrupt a good night's sleep.

Day Study Blend 1
1 tablespoon evening primrose oil
6 drops of rosemary
6 drops of basil
3 drops of lemon

Day Study Blend 2
1 tablespoon sweet almond oil
5 drops of grapefruit
5 drops of rosemary
4 drops of bergamot
1 drop of ginger

Day Study Blend 3
1 tablespoon sweet almond oil
5 drops of peppermint
5 drops of rosemary
5 drops of lemon

Day Study Blend 4
1 tablespoon sweet almond oil
10 drops of rosemary
2 drops of basil
2 drops of lavender
1 drop of grapefruit

Night Before Exam Blend 1
1 tablespoon evening primrose oil
6 drops of chamomile
4 drops of sandalwood
3 drops of geranium
2 drops of lavender

Night Before Exam Blend 2
1 tablespoon sweet almond
5 drops of marjoram
5 drops of lavender
5 drops of mandarin

❧ Bath Soak ❧

Blend all ingredients together and mix thoroughly. Apply to the bath water after the bath has been filled. Agitate the water to disperse the oils and soak for 20 minutes. The following recipes will make 1 treatment.

Refresh & Stimulate Blend 1
1 tablespoon sweet almond oil
5 drops of eucalyptus
5 drops of rosemary

Refresh & Stimulate Blend 2
1 tablespoon sweet almond oil
5 drops of basil
5 drops of lemon

Calm & Relaxation Blend 1
1 tablespoon sweet almond oil
5 drops of chamomile
5 drops of marjoram

Calm & Relaxation Blend 2
1 tablespoon sweet almond oil
5 drops of lavender
5 drops of sandalwood

❧ Diffuser/Oil Burner ❧

Place water and essential oils at the top of the diffuser and light the candle below. Light the candle 10 to 15 minutes before sitting down to study, to allow the aroma of the essential oils to fill the room. The following blends are not recommended for night time study as they stimulate the mind and could prevent a restful night's sleep.

Blend 1
8 drops of rosemary
4 drops of basil

Blend 2
5 drops of lemon
4 drops of peppermint
3 drops of rosemary

❧ Mist Sprays ❧

Blend all ingredients in a spray bottle and mix thoroughly. Spray over face, neck and chest, or around the immediate area several times during study. Always remember to inhale deeply. The following recipes should last 2 to 3 days, depending on the length and frequency of study periods.

Blend 1
30ml distilled water
15 drops of rosemary
10 drops of lemon
5 drops of basil

Blend 2
30ml distilled water
10 drops of grapefruit
10 drops of bergamot
5 drops of rosemary
5 drops of basil

Fatigue

Fatigue may occur for a variety of different reasons including lack of sleep, worry, stress, too much work, hormonal imbalance, poor diet, busy mind or an overactive lifestyle. While essential oils have the ability to make you feel more energetic, awake and fresh, the relief may only be short term if the fatigue is the result of an underlying health problem. It is therefore important to consult your doctor if the fatigue persists.

Essential oils for fatigue; Basil, Eucalyptus, Geranium, Lavender, Lemon, Lemongrass, Marjoram, Orange, Peppermint, Rosemary, Thyme.

Carrier oils for fatigue; Sweet Almond, Coconut, Grapeseed, Olive.

❧ Massage Oils ❧

Blend all ingredients together and mix thoroughly. Massage the formula into the upper chest, back of the neck, shoulders and arms. Because the oils used will have invigorating and uplifting properties, it is not recommended to use these recipes after 6pm as they have the potential to disturb a night's sleep. Repeat as and when is needed. The following recipes will yield enough for 1 treatment.

Blend 1
2 tablespoons sweet almond oil
8 drops of rosemary
4 drops of peppermint
3 drops of basil

Blend 2
2 tablespoons olive oil
6 drops of eucalyptus
5 drops of geranium
3 drops of lemon
1 drop of thyme

Blend 3
2 tablespoons melted coconut oil
5 drops of orange
4 drops of lavender
4 drops of lemon
2 drops of peppermint

Blend 4
2 tablespoons grapeseed oil
6 drops of eucalyptus
6 drops of geranium
3 drops of rosemary

❧ Diffuser/Oil Burner ❧

Place the water and essential oils at the top of the diffuser and light the candle below. Allow 10 to 15 minutes for the aroma to fill the room. Use the diffuser during the morning or afternoon, never in the evening due to the stimulating nature of the oils used.

Blend 1
4 drops of eucalyptus
4 drops of rosemary

Blend 2
6 drops of peppermint
2 drops of geranium

❧ Body Mist ❧

Blend all ingredients in a spray bottle and shake well to mix. Hold the bottle about 3 to 4 inches away from the upper body and spray liberally. Repeat this several times throughout the day as and when is needed. Do not spray after 6pm due to the stimulating nature of the oils used in these recipes. The following recipes will yield enough for approximately 2 days.

Blend 1
50ml distilled water
10 drops of peppermint
8 drops of rosemary
5 drops of geranium
2 drops of basil

Blend 2
50ml distilled water
8 drops of lemon
6 drops of geranium
4 drops of basil
4 drops of lavender
3 drops of rosemary

❧ Inhalations ❧

Inhaling essential oils from a tissue is an effective 'pick me up' whenever needed. Simply place your chosen drops of oils on a tissue and inhale throughout the day.

Blend 1
1 drop of peppermint
1 drop of eucalyptus

Blend 2
1 drop of geranium
1 drop of rosemary

Fever

A fever is an abnormally high temperature in the body, and is often accompanied by severe headaches, hot and cold sweats, muscle pain, sore throat, flu like symptoms, and sensitivity to light. It is usually a short term infection but can sometimes last for up to 3 weeks. Certain essential oils can ease some of the symptoms of fever but a medical consultation must always be undertaken.

Essential oils for fever; Basil, Black Pepper, Eucalyptus, Frankincense, Lemon.

Carrier oils for fever; Sweet Almond, Coconut, Grapeseed.

❧ Massage Oils ❧

Blend all ingredients together and mix thoroughly. Massage the formula into the chest, abdomen, back of the neck and bottoms of the feet. Repeat this 2 to 3 times per day. Allow the oils to absorb into the skin, do not wash off. Carry out each day until the fever subsides. The following recipes will yield enough for 1 day (2 treatments).

Blend 1	Blend 2
3 tablespoons coconut oil	3 tablespoons coconut oil
8 drops of peppermint	7 drops of lemon
7 drops of frankincense	7 drops of eucalyptus
5 drops of lemon	4 drops of peppermint
	2 drops of basil

❧ Body Mist ❧

Blend all ingredients together in a spray bottle and shake well to mix. Spray over the body several times per day and repeat daily until the fever subsides. Always shake well before use. The following recipes will yield enough for approximately 2 days.

Blend 1	Blend 2
60ml distilled water	60ml distilled water
15 drops of peppermint	10 drops of eucalyptus
5 drops of lemon	8 drops of frankincense
5 drops of basil	7 drops of peppermint

❧ Diffuser/Oil Burner ❧

Place the water and essential oils at the top of the diffuser and light the candle below. Allow 10 to 15 minutes for the aroma to fill the room. The following blends should only be used during the day as most oils in these recipes contain stimulating properties that may interfere with sleep.

Blend 1

6 drops of peppermint

Blend 2

4 drops of eucalyptus
2 drops of lemon

Flatulence

Flatulence is the passing of gas from the digestive system out of the anus. Commonly known as gas, flatulence can be an embarrassing problem for some people and is usually controlled by changes in the diet. When food or liquid is swallowed, small little pockets of air are also swallowed. Over time, this air builds up in the digestive system and needs to be released. The problem is exacerbated by eating foods that are difficult to digest, or by eating too quickly. Excessive flatulence can be related to an underlying health problem such as irritable bowel syndrome so it is very important to consult your doctor in this instance. Essential oils, when massaged into the abdomen can help to ease flatulence.

Essential oils for flatulence; Fennel, Ginger, Juniper, Lavender, Patchouli, Peppermint.

Carrier oils for flatulence; Sweet Almond, Coconut, Grapeseed, Olive.

❧ Massage Oils ❧

Blend all ingredients together and mix thoroughly. Gently massage the formula into the abdomen, in circular, clockwise movements. Repeat 2 to 3 times per day as and when is needed. Because peppermint is stimulating it is best to carry out this treatment in the morning or afternoon as it has the potential to disturb a night's sleep.

Blend 1
1 tablespoon grapeseed oil
4 drops of peppermint
4 drops of lavender
2 drops of fennel

Blend 2
1 tablespoon sweet almond oil
4 drops of patchouli
3 drops of peppermint
3 drops of ginger

Gingivitis

Gingivitis, also known as gum disease, is a very common disorder characterized by inflammation of the gums. It is caused by the build-up of plaque on the teeth and if not treated, a condition called periodontitis can develop which may cause tooth loss. Classic signs of gingivitis include red, inflamed, tender gums that may bleed during brushing. Good oral hygiene is essential to prevent this condition from occurring, however when it does, certain essential oils provide effective results in the treatment of gingivitis.

Essential oils for gingivitis; Chamomile (Roman), Clove, Eucalyptus, Lemon, Peppermint, Rosemary, Tea Tree, Thyme.

Carrier oils for gingivitis; Coconut, Aloe Vera (not a carrier oil as such but a very effective treatment for gingivitis).

❧ Mouth Rinse ❧

Add your chosen essential oils to a small cup of warm water. After brushing, swish well around the mouth for 40 to 60 seconds. Do NOT swallow the mouth rinse. Repeat each morning and before bedtime. The following recipes will yield enough for 1 treatment.

Blend 1
1 drop of tea tree
1 drop of clove
1 drop of lemon

Blend 2
1 drop of thyme
1 drop of lavender
1 drop of peppermint

❧ Toothpaste ❧

Add one drop of tea tree oil on top of the toothpaste before brushing. Do NOT swallow. Follow with a mouth rinse above.

❧ Gum Gel ❧

Mix ingredients thoroughly. Apply to the gums and leave for 1 to 2 minutes. Do NOT swallow. The following recipes will yield enough for 1 treatment.

Blend 1

½ teaspoon aloe vera gel
3 drops of tea tree

Blend 2

½ teaspoon aloe vera gel
2 drops of peppermint
1 drop of thyme

Hay Fever

Hay Fever is an allergic disorder of the membranes of the nose, throat and eyes. It is caused by increased sensitivity to airborne pollens, and is therefore usually seasonal. Hay fever is quite common and affects a large number of people, symptoms experienced may include itchy eyes, nose and throat, congestion, red and watery eyes, and sneezing, while coughing, breathlessness and wheezing often indicates the presence of allergic asthma also.

Essential oils which are generally helpful in treating allergies should always be given first choice in any treatment used to ease the condition. Massage is probably the most effective treatment as the oils are absorbed into the bloodstream and can directly oppose the offending allergen, also decreasing the severity of the allergic response.

Essential oils for hay fever; Chamomile (Roman), Eucalyptus, Lavender, Lemon, Marjoram, Melissa, Peppermint, Rosemary, Thyme.

Carrier oils for hay fever; Sweet Almond, Avocado, Coconut, Olive, Sesame.

❧ Massage Oils ❧

Blend all ingredients together and mix thoroughly. Gently massage the formula into the upper back and chest area. Carry out the massage first thing in the morning and repeat each night while the symptoms persist. The following recipes will yield enough for 1 treatment.

Blend 1
2 tablespoons grapeseed oil
5 drops of lavender
5 drops of chamomile
5 drops of rosemary
5 drops of lemon

Blend 2
2 tablespoons olive oil
10 drops of chamomile
4 drops of lemon
4 drops of lavender
2 drops of eucalyptus

Blend 3
2 tablespoons melted coconut oil
8 drops of eucalyptus
5 drops of lavender
4 drops of marjoram
3 drops of peppermint

Blend 4
2 tablespoons grapeseed oil
6 drops of lavender
5 drops of chamomile
5 drops of melissa
4 drops of eucalyptus

❧ Inhalations ❧

Caution should always be used when employing a steam inhalation as a form of treatment for hay fever, as heat can often worsen congestion, and many people end up feeling more uncomfortable as a result. A simple inhalation technique using a tissue is a very effective way to clear congestion. Simply place the appropriate drops of essential oils on a tissue and inhale throughout the day.

Blend 1
1 drop of peppermint
1 drop of lemon

Blend 2
1 drop of eucalyptus
1 drop of chamomile

Headaches

When essential oils are added to a bath or massaged into the body, they are infused into the bloodstream and can act as a natural painkiller. The key to a successful remedy for headaches using aromatherapy is remembering that less is more. Essential oils are highly concentrated oils with strong aromas and can worsen a headache if overused. Never exceed 5 drops in any blend.

Essential oils for headaches; Chamomile (Roman), Clary Sage, Eucalyptus, Lavender, Peppermint, Rosemary, Thyme.

Carrier oils for headaches; Sweet Almond Oil, Apricot Kernel, Avocado, Coconut.

❧ Treatment Oils ❧

Blend all ingredients together and mix thoroughly. Massage several drops of the formula into the forehead, temples and back of the neck each time you suffer from a headache. The following recipes will yield enough for 1 treatment. Some headache sufferers may find the aroma of essential oils too over powering in which case it is not recommended to carry out this treatment.

Blend 1
1 tablespoon avocado oil
2 drops of lavender
2 drops of peppermint

Blend 2
1 tablespoon sweet almond oil
4 drops of lavender
1 drop of eucalyptus

Blend 3
1 tablespoon coconut oil
2 drops of rosemary
2 drops of eucalyptus

Blend 4
1 tablespoon apricot kernel
1 drop of rosemary
1 drop of clary sage
1 drop of lavender
1 drop of peppermint

❧ Treatment Compress ❧

Placing an essential oil compress across the forehead can be a helpful way to ease the discomfort of a headache. It is also effective if you cover the back of the neck with a compress.

Fill a large bowl with cold water, add the essential oils, agitate the water to disperse the oils, soak the compress for 2 minutes, wring out excess water and apply to the forehead or back of the neck (2 can be applied at the same time on both the forehead and neck). Sit and relax for 20 minutes.

Blend 1
1 large bowl of water
4 drops of lavender
1 drop of peppermint

Blend 2
1 large bowl of water
3 drops of clary sage
2 drops of chamomile

Blend 3
1 large bowl of water
4 drops of rosemary
1 drop of thyme

Blend 4
1 large bowl of water
2 drops of eucalyptus
2 drops of thyme
1 drop of lavender

Hemorrhoids

A hemorrhoid, or piles as they are more commonly known, is a condition in which the veins around the anus are abnormally dilated. The causes may be various but a common factor is restriction of the normal circulation of blood to the rectum. This may occur temporarily during pregnancy, due to the pressure of the uterus, or the condition may be continually present due to disease of the liver or chronic constipation. Other causes are said to be lack of dietary fiber, straining at stool, obesity, heaving lifting, athletic exertions or constant sitting. Bleeding, irritation and itching and common symptoms. Treatment should be aimed at improving circulation generally, as well as treating locally.

Essential oils for hemorrhoids; Chamomile (Roman), Cypress, Fennel, Frankincense, Geranium, Juniper, Lavender, Lemon, Marjoram, Peppermint, Rosemary, Tea Tree.

Carrier oils for hemorrhoids; Sweet Almond, Avocado, Coconut, Evening Primrose, Grapeseed, Olive.

❧ Massage Oils ❧

Blend all ingredients together and mix thoroughly. In this instance massage is used to stimulate digestion and help eradicate constipation should that be a problem. Massage the formula into the abdomen in a circular clockwise motion. Leave the oils to absorb into the skin, do not wash off. The following recipes will yield enough for 1 treatment. Repeat everyday for as long as is needed.

Blend 1
1 tablespoon grapeseed oil
5 drops of rosemary
3 drops of marjoram
2 drops of fennel

Blend 2
1 tablespoon sweet almond oil
4 drops of lemon
2 drops of ginger
2 drops of peppermint
2 drops of basil

❧ Sitz Bath Oils ❧

Fill the bath with warm water (not hot), running the water until it reaches waist level. Add the essential oils and any other ingredients to the bath once it has been filled. Agitate the water to disperse the oils. Soak for 20 to 30 minutes. Immediately after the bath, have a cold shower to regulate circulation.

Blend 1
1 tablespoon olive oil
6 drops of juniper
6 drops of peppermint

Blend 2
4 tablespoons witch hazel
8 drops of lavender
4 drops of cypress

❧ Cold Compress ❧

Prepare a bowl of cold water and add your chosen essential oils. Place the compress into the water and allow to soak for 2 minutes. Remove and wring out any excess water. Apply over the affected area and leave for 20 minutes. Each time the compress starts to warm to body heat, dip back into the water to refresh it. Suitable for external hemorrhoids only.

Blend 1
½ cup apple cider vinegar
2 drops of lavender
2 drops of juniper
1 drop of tea tree
1 drop of marjoram

Blend 2
4 tablespoons fresh lemon juice
3 drops of geranium
3 drops of cypress

Blend 3
½ cup apple cider vinegar
2 drops of peppermint
2 drops of juniper
2 drops of geranium

Blend 4
4 drops of cypress
1 drop of lemon
1 drop of tea tree

Indigestion

Indigestion is a pain or discomfort in the chest or stomach that is triggered by food or liquid and usually occurs soon after food or drink has been consumed. It is a common digestive disorder that can occur in people of all ages, and is usually caused by stomach acid breaking down the mucosa of the digestive tract. Typical symptoms of indigestion include heartburn, bloating, chest pain or belching. Certain medications, stress, smoking, obesity and pregnancy can also cause indigestion.

Essential oils for indigestion; Chamomile (Roman), Fennel, Ginger, Juniper, Lemon, Lemongrass, Orange, Patchouli, Peppermint.

Carrier oils for indigestion; Coconut, Grapeseed, Olive.

❧ Massage Oils ❧

Blend all ingredients together and mix thoroughly. Apply the formula to the abdomen and gently massage using circular clockwise movements around the abdomen area. Repeat each day until the digestive system normalizes and symptoms ease. The following recipes will yield enough for 1 treatment.

Blend 1
1 tablespoon grapeseed oil
8 drops of peppermint
2 drops of lavender

Blend 2
1 tablespoon olive oil
4 drops of orange
3 drops of chamomile
3 drops of peppermint

Blend 3
1 tablespoon coconut oil
5 drops of orange
5 drops of chamomile

Blend 4
1 tablespoon grapeseed oil
4 drops of lemon
3 drops of peppermint
2 drops of fennel
1 drop of ginger

Insomnia

Stressful situations, busy lifestyles, restlessness, depression and sickness are just some of the root causes of this frustrating disorder. Over a long period of time, insomnia can have a negative impact on our well being and the overall quality of our lives. Thankfully many essential oils have calming, sedative properties that will enable you to relax, calm your mind and enter a deep sleep.

Essential oils for insomnia; Chamomile (Roman), Clary Sage, Mandarin, Marjoram, Neroli, Petitgrain, Rose, Sandalwood, Valerian, Vetiver.

Carrier oils for insomnia; Sweet Almond, Apricot Kernel, Coconut, Evening Primrose, Wheatgerm.

❧ Massage Oils ❧

Blend all ingredients together and mix thoroughly. Apply to the entire body or massage into the chest, neck, shoulders and arms just before bedtime. Leave the oils to absorb into the skin. If you are following up this treatment with a bath, leave the oils on for 30 minutes and have your bath (do not rub the oils off). Repeat each night before bedtime. The following recipes will yield enough for 1 treatment.

Blend 1
2 tablespoons coconut oil
6 drops of marjoram
6 drops of lavender
6 drops of chamomile
2 drops of neroli

Blend 2
2 tablespoons sweet almond oil
6 drops of valerian
4 drops of sandalwood
4 drops of vetiver
4 drops of lavender
2 drops of marjoram

Blend 3
2 tablespoons evening primrose oil
10 drops of clary sage
5 drops of chamomile
5 drops of vetiver

Blend 4
2 tablespoons coconut oil
10 drops of lavender
10 drops of chamomile

❧ Treatment Baths ❧

Blend all ingredients together and mix thoroughly. Add to the bath once it has been filled. Agitate the water to disperse the oils. Soak for 20 minutes. Repeat each night before bedtime.

Blend 1
1 tablespoon sweet almond oil
5 drops of lavender

Blend 2
1 tablespoon coconut oil
2 drops of vetiver
2 drops of sandalwood
1 drop of lavender

Blend 3
1 tablespoon olive oil
3 drops of chamomile
2 drops of valerian

Blend 4
1 tablespoon evening primrose oil
2 drops of marjoram
2 drops of lavender

Itching

Itching is a very common condition that can be extremely annoying and frustrating for the individual concerned. There are many different causes associated with itching including eczema, psoriasis, insect bites, dry skin, allergic reactions, or even soaps and detergents. Essential oils with anti-inflammatory and soothing properties have the ability to provide relief to itchy skin and alleviate any irritation.

Essential oils for itching; Basil, Chamomile (Roman), Clove, Frankincense, Geranium, Juniper, Lavender, Lemon, Neroli, Peppermint, Rosemary.

Carrier oils for itching; Sweet Almond, Avocado, Borage Seed, Coconut, Evening Primrose, Grapeseed, Jojoba, Aloe Vera (not a carrier oil as such but a very effective treatment for itching).

❧ Massage Oils ❧

Blend all ingredients together and mix thoroughly. Massage the formula into the affected area and leave the oils to absorb into the skin. Repeat twice daily, once in the morning and again in the evening, until your skin normalizes. The following recipes will yield enough for 1 treatment on a specific area. If you are massaging the entire body, double the drops of essential oils and use 3 tablespoons of carrier oil.

Blend 1
1 tablespoon sweet almond oil
1 teaspoon evening primrose
6 drops of peppermint
3 drops of chamomile
1 drop of lavender

Blend 2
1 tablespoon coconut oil
1 teaspoon aloe vera gel
5 drops of frankincense
5 drops of lavender

Blend 3
1 tablespoon borage seed oil
1 teaspoon evening primrose oil
4 drops of juniper
4 drops of geranium
2 drops of peppermint

Blend 4
1 tablespoon avocado oil
1 teaspoon coconut oil
4 drops of neroli
3 drops of lavender
3 drops of juniper

❧ Bath Oils ❧

Blend all ingredients together, mix thoroughly and add to water once the bath has been filled. Ensure that the bath water is lukewarm, hot water may irritate the itching further. Agitate the water to disperse the oils and soak for 15 to 20 minutes.

Blend 1
1 tablespoon fractionated coconut oil
4 drops of rosemary
3 drops of geranium
3 drops of peppermint

Blend 2
1 tablespoon sweet almond oil
6 drops of peppermint
4 drops of frankincense

❧ Body Mist ❧

Blend all ingredients together in a spray bottle and shake well to mix. Holding the bottle about 3 to 4 inches away from the affected area, spray liberally. Repeat several times throughout the day as soon as you feel your skin starting to become irritated. The following recipes will yield enough for approximately 2 days, depending on the size of the area being treated.

Blend 1
50ml distilled water
8 drops of peppermint
6 drops of lavender
6 drops of chamomile

Blend 2
50ml distilled water
10 drops of frankincense
6 drops of lavender
4 drops of rosemary
1 drop of chamomile

Jet Lag

Jet lag is unfortunately something we cannot avoid when travelling long distances by air. When we travel across time zones, our body's internal clock experiences a natural disturbance and, as a result, fatigue and disorientation set in. Swollen ankles and sleep disturbance are also common symptoms. Essential oils are a very effective treatment for the symptoms of jet lag and should be prepared before the journey.

Essential oils for jet lag; Bergamot, Chamomile (Roman), Clary Sage, Cypress, Eucalyptus, Geranium, Grapefruit, Juniper, Lavender, Lemon, Mandarin, Marjoram, Peppermint, Rosemary.

Carrier oils for jet lag; Sweet Almond, Avocado, Coconut, Grapeseed, Olive, Sesame.

❧ Massage Oils ❧

Blend all ingredients together and mix thoroughly. Massage the formula into the chest, shoulders, back of the neck and both arms. If you arrive to your destination in the morning, use the uplifting, enliven blends. If you arrive in the evening however, use the relaxing, calming blends to help you drift off into a peaceful sleep. Use the swollen ankles blend when you arrive at your destination.

Relax & Calm Blend 1
2 tablespoons grapeseed oil
6 drops of lavender
6 drops of chamomile
3 drops of mandarin

Relax & Calm Blend 2
2 tablespoons coconut oil
5 drops of marjoram
5 drops of clary sage
5 drops of lavender

Uplift & Enliven Blend 1
2 tablespoons olive oil
6 drops of grapefruit
5 drops of rosemary
4 drops of bergamot

Uplift & Enliven Blend 2
2 tablespoons grapeseed oil
8 drops of lemon
4 drops of eucalyptus
3 drops of rosemary

Swollen Ankles Blend
1 tablespoon grapeseed oil
6 drops of cypress
4 drops of juniper

Mental Clarity Blend
1 tablespoon coconut oil
4 drops of clary sage
3 drops of basil
3 drops of rosemary

❧ Bath Oils ❧

Blend all ingredients together and mix thoroughly. Add the blend to bath water, once the bath has been filled. Agitate the water to disperse the oils and soak for 15 to 20 minutes. Use the relaxing blend if you arrive at your destination in the evening, this will help you to relax and drift off into a good night's sleep. If you arrive in the morning or early afternoon, the uplift and enliven blend will energize and awaken the senses so you can stay awake throughout the day. For swollen ankles, prepare a basin of warm water and soak the feet for 10 minutes.

Relax & Calm Blend
1 tablespoon olive oil
8 drops of lavender
2 drops of chamomile

Uplift & Enliven Blend
1 tablespoon olive oil
6 drops of lemon
4 drops of eucalyptus

Swollen Ankles Blend
2 tablespoons Epsom salts
3 drops of cypress
3 drops of grapefruit

❧ Body Mist ❧

Blend all ingredients in a spray bottle and shake well to mix. Spray on the body throughout the day to help keep you feeling awake and fresh. To sleep at night, you can either spray on the body before bed, or use as a pillow mist.

Enliven & Uplifting Blend
50ml distilled water
5 drops of lemongrass
5 drops of juniper
5 drops of rosemary

Mental Clarity Blend
50ml distilled water
6 drops of lemon
4 drops of rosemary
3 drops of peppermint
2 drops of geranium

Relax & Calm Blend
50ml distilled water
5 drops of neroli
5 drops of chamomile
5 drops of marjoram

Leg Cramps

Leg cramps are a common condition where the muscles in the leg become tight and painful. These are sudden, involuntary contractions that can last up to a few seconds or, in more severe cases, several minutes. The cramp quite often occurs in the calf muscle, although it can affect any part of the leg, including feet and back of the thighs. It is also common that you may experience pain and tenderness in your leg for several hours after the cramp has passed. Cramps can occur for a variety of reasons including tired or overworked muscles, insufficient mineral supply to the muscle, flat feet, dehydration or ill fitting shoes. People of all ages can be affected by this condition but it is more common in adults over 60. It is also common during pregnancy. Essential oils that are natural muscle relaxers, plus those that have anti-inflammatory and analgesic properties are an effective treatment for leg cramps.

Essential oils for leg cramps; Basil, Chamomile (Roman), Clove, Cypress, Ginger, Lavender, Lemongrass, Marjoram, Peppermint, Rosemary.

Carrier oils for leg cramps; Avocado, Coconut, Grapeseed, Olive.

❧ Massage Oils ❧

Blend all ingredients together and mix thoroughly. Massage the formula into the entire leg, working in an upwards motion towards the heart. Finish off by massaging the foot. Carry out this treatment twice per day, once in the morning and once at night. Because leg cramps are common during sleep it is important to apply the formula just before bedtime. However because some oils in the following recipes have stimulating properties, you may find they interfere with your sleep, in which case carry out the 2nd treatment late afternoon. The following recipes will yield enough for 1 treatment.

Blend 1
1 tablespoon coconut oil
4 drops of rosemary
3 drops of lavender
3 drops of marjoram

Blend 2
1 tablespoon grapeseed oil
5 drops of peppermint
4 drops of chamomile
1 drop of ginger

Blend 3

1 tablespoon olive oil

4 drops of lemongrass

3 drops of marjoram

3 drops of peppermint

Blend 4

1 tablespoon grapeseed oil

5 drops of marjoram

3 drops of lavender

2 drops of cypress

Memory Loss

Memory loss is a condition that most people experience at some point in their lives. The older we get, however, the more likely it is for us to have longer and more regular bouts of memory loss. Certain essential oils can help to enhance memory, improve concentration and focus, and help to create mental clarity.

Essential oils for memory loss; Basil, Grapefruit, Ginger, Jasmine, Lemon, Neroli, Rose, Rosemary, Thyme.

Carrier oils for memory loss; Sweet Almond, Avocado, Coconut, Olive, Sesame.

❧ Massage Oils ❧

Blend all ingredients together and mix thoroughly. Massage the formula into the chest, shoulders, back and front of the neck, and both arms. Leave the oils to absorb, do not wash off. Carry out this treatment once per day, preferably in the mornings. Repeat every day. The following recipes will yield enough for 1 treatment.

Blend 1	Blend 2
2 tablespoons coconut oil	2 tablespoons grapeseed oil
8 drops of rosemary	5 drops of jasmine
4 drops of basil	5 drops of lemon
3 drops of grapefruit	5 drops of rosemary

❧ Diffuser/Oil Burner ❧

Place the water and essential oils at the top of the diffuser and light the candle below. Allow 10 to 15 minutes for the aroma to fill the room. Repeat this for a couple of hours in the morning or afternoon when you feel the need.

Blend 1	Blend 2
6 drops of rosemary	4 drops of basil
	2 drops of jasmine

Menopause

Menopause is triggered by decreasing hormones and is a significant change in a woman's life, both physically and emotionally. Common symptoms include hot flushes, day and night sweats, mood swings, accelerated signs of ageing and water retention and bloating. Aromatherapy can help with both the physiological and psychological aspects of menopause.

Essential oils for menopause; Bergamot, Chamomile (Roman), Clary Sage, Cypress, Geranium, Jasmine, Lemon, Fennel (Sweet), Grapefruit.

Carrier oils for menopause; Sweet Almond, Apricot Kernel, Coconut, Evening Primrose, Grapeseed, Jojoba, Wheatgerm.

❧ Massage Oils ❧

Blend all ingredients together and mix thoroughly. Massage the whole body or smaller areas like the chest, arms, legs or abdomen. Repeat daily. The following recipes will yield enough for 1 treatment on the entire body.

Hot Flushes Blend
3 tablespoons grapeseed oil
8 drops of peppermint
8 drops of geranium
8 drops of chamomile

Day & Night Sweats Blend
3 tablespoons evening primrose oil
8 drops of grapefruit
8 drops of lemon
8 drops of jasmine

Water Retention & Bloating Blend
3 tablespoons coconut oil
10 drops of lemon
6 drops of fennel
6 drops of cypress

Mood Lifting Blend
3 tablespoons sweet almond oil
5 drops of neroli
5 drops of mandarin
5 drops of bergamot
5 drops of clary sage

❧ Bath Blends ❧

Blend all ingredients together and mix thoroughly. Add to the water in the bath, agitate the water so the oils disperse. Soak for 20 minutes. Repeat daily.

Hot Flush Blend
1 tablespoon sweet almond oil
10 drops of peppermint
2 drops of lavender

Day & Night Sweats Blend
1 tablespoon coconut oil
6 drops of peppermint
6 drops of lemon
2 drops of grapefruit

Water Retention & Bloating Blend
1 tablespoon grapeseed oil
8 drops of peppermint
6 drops of fennel

Mood Lifting Blend
1 tablespoon grapeseed oil
4 drops of sandalwood
2 drops of geranium
2 drops of rosemary
2 drops of lemon

❧ Body & Face Spritz ❧

Spraying a cool, refreshing spritz on the face or body is a perfect way to cool down during a hot flush or during day and night sweats. When you go out, keep the bottle in your bag, and as soon as you feel a hot flush coming on, hold the bottle about 4 inches from the face, close your eyes and spray liberally. Repeat as often as is needed.

Hot Flush Blend
50ml distilled water
15 drops of peppermint

Day & Night Sweats Blend
50ml distilled water
6 drops of clary sage
5 drops of lavender
4 drops of bergamot

Mood Lifting Blend 1
50ml distilled water
10 drops of clary sage
10 drops of bergamot

Mood Lifting Blend 2
50ml rosewater
8 drops of lavender
8 drops of rosemary

4 drops of geranium

❧ Bath Salts ❧

Epsom salts are a fantastic choice for a relaxing bath as they are rich in magnesium, an excellent muscle relaxant and sedative for the nervous system. Add the Epsom salts first, and then fill the bath. Once the water is ready, add the oil blend and agitate the water to disperse the oils. Soak for 20 minutes. Repeat 2-3 times each week before bedtime.

Blend 1
1 cup Epsom salts
1 tablespoon olive oil
5 drops of lavender
5 drops of vetiver

Blend 2
1 cup Epsom salts
1 tablespoon evening primrose oil
5 drops of chamomile
5 drops of valerian

❧ Pillow Spritz ❧

Place all ingredients in a spray bottle and shake well to mix. Each night before you lie down, hold the nozzle about 3-4 inches from the pillow, and spray 4-5 times around the entire surface. Repeat each night. Shake well before use.

Blend 1
30ml distilled water
15 drops of lavender

Blend 2
30ml chamomile hydrosol
5 drops of valerian
5 drops of marjoram
5 drops of neroli

Blend 3
30ml lavender hydrosol
10 drops of chamomile
5 drops of vetiver

Blend 4
30ml distilled water
8 drops of vetiver
8 drops of chamomile

❧ Vaporizer/Oil Burner ❧

Place a vaporizer/oil burner in your bedroom about 6 feet away from the bed ensuring that it is on a safe surface. Add the water followed by the essential oils at the top, and burn a candle at the bottom. Light the candle about 30 minutes before you go to bed to allow the relaxing aroma to fill the room.

Blend 1
5 drops of lavender

Blend 2
5 drops of chamomile

Blend 3
5 drops of vetiver

Blend 4
2 drops of lavender
2 drops of chamomile
1 drop of valerian

Menstrual Cramps

Caused by contractions of the uterus during menstruation, menstrual cramps are a painful condition and are often accompanied by nausea, headaches and backache. Essential oils that help to balance the hormones and provide pain relief are the best choice of oils to use.

Essential oils for menstrual cramps; Basil, Chamomile (Roman), Clary Sage, Fennel, Jasmine, Geranium, Lavender, Marjoram, Peppermint, Rosemary, Valerian, Vetiver.

Carrier oils for menstrual cramps; Sweet Almond, Coconut, Evening Primrose, Grapeseed, Olive.

❧ Massage Oils ❧

Blend all ingredients together and mix thoroughly. Massage in a clockwise motion around the abdomen and lower back. Apply when needed. Leave the oils to absorb into the skin, do not wash off. The following recipes will yield enough for 1 treatment.

Blend 1
2 tablespoons sweet almond oil
8 drops of clary sage
5 drops of marjoram
2 drops of lavender

Blend 2
2 tablespoons evening primrose
3 drops of clary sage
3 drops of fennel
3 drops of lavender
3 drops of marjoram
3 drops of jasmine

Blend 3
2 tablespoons coconut oil
6 drops of peppermint
6 drops of lavender
3 drops of cypress

Blend 4
2 tablespoons evening primrose oil
5 drops of chamomile
5 drops of clary sage
5 drops of geranium

❧ Hot Compress ❧

Soak the compress in a bowl of hot water and your chosen essential oils for 2 minutes to allow the oils to absorb into the compress. Remove, wring out any excess water and apply across the abdomen (make sure the compress is not too hot so as to avoid burning the skin). Repeat daily throughout menstruation.

Blend 1

8 drops of marjoram
6 drops of clary sage
2 drops of lavender

Blend 2

6 drops of peppermint
4 drops of lavender
4 drops of chamomile
2 drops of marjoram

Migraines

A migraine attack is believed to begin with spasm of the arteries, causing the visual and neurological symptoms, followed by arterial dilation, causing the headache. The headache becomes throbbing in character and is often accompanied by nausea and vomiting. Headaches tend to last for several hours and may persist for days. Aromatherapy is better used as a preventative measure rather than an attempted treatment for migraine. Once a migraine attack has begun many sufferers are unable to tolerate the smell of essential oils or anybody touching their heads. Extremely light massage of the temples might be helpful if touching the head does not make the pain worse.

Essential oils for migraines; Lavender, Marjoram, Peppermint.

Carrier oils for migraines; Sweet Almond, Coconut, Jojoba.

❧ Cold Compress ❧

Prepare a bowl of cold water and add your chosen essential oils. Place the compress into the water and allow to soak for 2 minutes. Remove and wring out any excess water. Apply the compress across the forehead, sit back and relax for 20 minutes, preferably in the dark. Each time the compress starts to warm to body heat, dip back into the water to refresh it.

Blend 1
6 drops of lavender

Blend 2
3 drops of lavender
3 drops of peppermint

❧ Massage Oils ❧

Blend all ingredients together and mix thoroughly. Gently massage the formula into the temples, forehead and neck. Some migraine sufferers may only be able to carry out this treatment at the very beginning of an attack because of their intolerance to smells. The following recipes will yield enough for 1 treatment.

Blend 1
1 teaspoon coconut oil
2 drops of chamomile
1 drop of lavender

Blend 2
1 teaspoon sweet almond
2 drops of neroli
1 drop of lemon

❧ Diffuser/Oil Burner ❧

Place the water and essential oils at the top of the diffuser and light the candle below. Allow 10 to 15 minutes for the aroma to fill the room. This is an excellent preventative measure but can also be used during a migraine attack if the sufferer can tolerate the scent.

Blend 1
1 drop of lavender
1 drop of chamomile
1 drop of neroli

Blend 2
2 drops of lemon
1 drop of peppermint

Muscular Aches & Pains

Muscular aches & pains can occur due to a number of different reasons such as over-exercising, bad posture, PMS, sickness, or fibromyalgia. When it comes to pain relief, there are many essential oils to choose from. Ones that contain analgesic (pain relief), anti-inflammatory and anti-rheumatic properties are the best choice.

Essential oils for muscular aches & pains; Basil, Chamomile (Roman), Clary Sage, Cypress, Eucalyptus, Frankincense, Ginger, Juniper Berry, Lavender, Marjoram, Peppermint, Rosemary, Sandalwood, Thyme, Vetiver.

Carrier oils for muscular aches & pains; Sweet Almond, Apricot Kernel, Coconut, Grapeseed, Wheatgerm.

❧ Massage Oils ❧

Blend all ingredients together and mix thoroughly. Massage the formula into tight or stiff muscles, along with the surrounding area. Repeat as and when is needed. The following recipes will yield enough for 1 treatment.

Blend 1
2 tablespoons grapeseed oil
10 drops of rosemary
3 drops of juniper
2 drops of lavender

Blend 2
2 tablespoons sweet almond oil
6 drops of chamomile
5 drops of eucalyptus
2 drops of ginger
2 drops of marjoram

Blend 3
2 tablespoons apricot kernel oil
5 drops of peppermint
5 drops of clary sage
5 drops of lavender

Blend 4
2 tablespoons coconut oil
8 drops of eucalyptus
4 drops of vetiver
3 drops of cypress

❧ Bath Oils ❧

Blend all ingredients together and mix thoroughly. Add the formula to the bath water and agitate until the oils have dispersed. Soak for 20 minutes.

Blend 1
1 tablespoon sweet almond oil
10 drops of peppermint
10 drops of marjoram
5 drops of chamomile

Blend 2
1 tablespoon wheatgerm oil
10 drops of juniper berry
10 drops of eucalyptus
2 drops of thyme
2 drops of lavender

Blend 3
1 tablespoon apricot kernel
5 drops of marjoram
5 drops of sandalwood
5 drops of frankincense
5 drops of basil

Blend 4
1 tablespoon coconut oil
15 drops of chamomile
10 drops of lavender

❧ Bath Salts ❧

Add the Epsom salts to the bath before the water. Once the bath has been filled, add the essential oils and agitate the water to disperse the salt and oils. Soak for 20 minutes.

Blend 1
2 cups Epsom salts
1 tablespoon grapeseed oil
4 drops of eucalyptus
4 drops of peppermint
4 drops of rosemary
4 drops of thyme

Blend 2
2 cups of Epsom salts
1 tablespoon coconut oil
8 drops of chamomile
4 drops of marjoram
4 drops of lavender

Muscular Stiffness

Muscles generally become tight and stiff after exercise, repetitive motion or prolonged periods of inactivity. Essential oil treatments incorporating massage and hot baths can help to relieve muscles, increasing suppleness and flexibility.

Essential oils for stiff, tight muscles; Basil, Cedarwood, Chamomile (Roman), Clary Sage, Cypress, Eucalyptus, Geranium, Lavender, Lemon, Lemongrass, Marjoram, Peppermint, Rosemary.

Carrier oils for stiff, tight muscles; Sweet Almond, Avocado, Coconut, Grapeseed.

❧ Massage Oils ❧

Blend all ingredients together and mix thoroughly. Massage the formula into tight or stiff muscles, along with the surrounding area. Repeat as and when is needed. The following recipes will yield enough for 1 treatment.

Blend 1
2 tablespoons sweet almond oil
10 drops of marjoram
5 drops of eucalyptus
5 drops of chamomile

Blend 2
2 tablespoons coconut oil
10 drops of lavender
10 drops of peppermint

Blend 3
2 tablespoons grapeseed oil
8 drops of cypress
8 drops of clary sage
4 drops of marjoram

Blend 4
2 tablespoons avocado oil
5 drops of chamomile
5 drops of lavender
5 drops of clary sage
5 drops of peppermint

❧ Bath Oils ❧

Blend all ingredients together and mix thoroughly. Add the formula to the bath water and agitate until the oils have dispersed. Soak for 20 minutes.

Blend 1

1 tablespoon sweet almond oil

10 drops of eucalyptus

5 drops of rosemary

Blend 2

1 tablespoon evening primrose oil

5 drops of cedarwood

5 drops of chamomile

5 drops of lemongrass

Blend 3

1 tablespoon sweet almond oil

8 drops of eucalyptus

4 drops of peppermint

3 drops of lemon

Blend 4

1 tablespoon evening primrose oil

10 drops of marjoram

2 drops of peppermint

2 drops of rosemary

1 drop of lavender

❧ Bath Salts ❧

Add the Epsom salts to the bath before the water. Once the bath has been filled, add the essential oils and agitate the water to disperse the salt and oils. Soak for 20 minutes.

Blend 1

2 cups Epsom salts

1 tablespoon grapeseed oil

10 drops of marjoram

2 drops of eucalyptus

2 drops of clary sage

2 drops of lavender

Blend 2

2 cups Epsom salts

1 tablespoon olive oil

8 drops of cypress

4 drops of chamomile

4 drops of lemongrass

Nausea & Vomiting

Nausea and/or vomiting can occur for a variety of different reasons including food poisoning, migraines, menstrual cramps, motion sickness, stomach flu, and morning sickness (usually during the 1ˢᵗ trimester of pregnancy in which case essential oils should never be used). Essential oils are quite an effective treatment for mild to moderate cases of nausea and/or vomiting, a more severe case can be the sign of a more serious health issue, your doctor should be consulted in this instance.

Essential oils for nausea & vomiting; Basil, Chamomile (Roman), Fennel, Ginger, Lavender, Peppermint, Rose, Sandalwood.

Carrier oils for nausea & vomiting; Coconut, Grapeseed, Olive.

❧ Body Mist ❧

Blend all ingredients together in a spray bottle and shake well to mix. Hold the bottle about 3 to 4 inches away from face and upper body, and spray each time you feel a pang of nausea. Some people may find that the aroma of essential oils makes them feel worse, in which case the use of essential oils is not recommended. The following recipes will yield enough for 1 day.

Blend 1
50ml distilled water
6 drops of peppermint
3 drops of lavender
1 drop of ginger

Blend 2
50ml distilled water
4 drops of lavender
4 drops of chamomile
2 drops of basil

❧ Massage Oils ❧

Blend all ingredients together and mix thoroughly. Apply the massage formula to the abdomen and gently massage this area using circular, clockwise movements. Carry out this treatment first thing in the morning and continue with a body spray (recipes above) throughout your day. The following recipes will yield enough for 1 treatment.

Blend 1

1 tablespoon grapeseed oil
4 drops of peppermint
1 drop of chamomile
1 drop of ginger

Blend 2

1 tablespoon coconut oil
3 drops of peppermint
2 drops of lavender
1 drop of basil

❧ Diffuser/Oil Burner ❧

Place the water and essential oils at the top of the diffuser and light the candle below. Allow 10 to 15 minutes for the aroma to fill the room. The following blends should only be used during the day as some oils used are stimulants and, as a result, may disrupt sleep.

Blend 1

5 drops of peppermint

Blend 2

3 drops of lavender
1 drop of basil
1 drop of peppermint

❧ Inhalations ❧

A simple inhalation technique using a tissue is an effective form of nausea relief. Each time you feel a wave of nausea, inhale the essential oils from the tissue.

Blend 1

2 drops of peppermint

Blend 2

1 drop of lavender
1 drop of ginger

Post Exercise

Varying degrees of muscle stiffness and soreness are often typical after a workout and can be a painful experience for some people. Essential oils provide natural pain relief, they help to relieve inflammation, and also help to reduce the stress that is often associated with muscular aches and pains.

Essential oils for post exercise; Benzoin, Black Pepper, Chamomile (Roman), Eucalyptus, Ginger, Juniper, Lavender, Lemon, Marjoram, Peppermint, Rosemary.

Carrier oils for post exercise; Coconut, Grapeseed, Hazelnut, Olive, Sesame.

❧ Massage Oils ❧

Blend all ingredients together and mix thoroughly. Massage the formula into tight, sore muscles along with the surrounding areas. Repeat 2 to 3 days after the workout. Leave to absorb into the skin, do not wash off. The following recipes will yield enough for 1 treatment.

Blend 1
1 tablespoon sesame oil
1 tablespoon olive oil
10 drops of eucalyptus
8 drops of juniper
2 drops of lemon

Blend 2
2 tablespoons grapeseed oil
2 drops of marjoram
6 drops of lavender
6 drops of peppermint
2 drops of rosemary

Blend 3
2 tablespoons grapeseed oil
5 drops of lemon
5 drops of eucalyptus
5 drops of peppermint
3 drops of rosemary
2 drops of ginger

Blend 4
2 tablespoons borage seed oil
10 drops of marjoram
6 drops of peppermint
4 drops of ginger

❧ Bath Oils ❧

Add the Epsom salts to the bath before the water. Once the bath has been filled, add the essential oils blend, agitate the water to disperse the oils and soak for 20 minutes.

Blend 1

2 cups Epsom salts
1 tablespoon olive oil
5 drops of marjoram
5 drops of eucalyptus
5 drops of lemon

Blend 2

2 cups Epsom salts
1 tablespoon grapeseed oil
6 drops of rosemary
6 drops of juniper
3 drops of peppermint

Pre Exercise

Before every workout, whether it is a gym class or ball game, it is vitally important to warm up the body to prepare muscles for exercise, in order to prevent strain or injury. Essential oils are an excellent way to enhance any workout by keeping the body hydrated, increasing mental focus, reducing fatigue and muscle pain, and helping with inflammation.

Essential oils for pre exercise; Eucalyptus, Frankincense, Ginger, Grapefruit, Lavender, Lemongrass, Peppermint, Rosemary.

Carrier oils for pre exercise; Sweet Almond, Borage Seed, Coconut, Grapeseed, Sesame.

❧ Massage Oils ❧

Blend all ingredients together and mix thoroughly. About 20 minutes before a workout, massage the formula into the muscles, concentrating on the larger muscle groups such as the quadriceps and hamstrings. Also make sure to massage the shoulders and arms. Leave to absorb into the skin, do not wash off. The following recipes will yield enough for 1 treatment.

Blend 1
2 tablespoons grapeseed oil
8 drops of peppermint
8 drops of rosemary
4 drops of lavender

Blend 2
2 tablespoons borage seed oil
6 drops of eucalyptus
6 drops of frankincense
5 drops of ginger
3 drops of lavender

Blend 3
2 tablespoons melted coconut oil
5 drops of grapefruit
5 drops of peppermint
4 drops of lavender
4 drops of ginger
2 drops of eucalyptus

Blend 4
2 tablespoons grapeseed oil
10 drops of peppermint
5 drops of rosemary
5 drops of lavender

Pre Menstrual Tension

Pre menstrual tension or pre menstrual syndrome, PMT or PMS as it is better known, is a hormonal imbalance in the body in the days leading up to menstruation. Fluid retention, breast swelling and tenderness, irritability, frustration, anger, anxiety, aches & pains and mood swings are just some of the symptoms. Thankfully certain essential oils have proven extremely effective at treating these symptoms and can be used in a variety of different ways.

Because every woman is different, it is difficult to set an exact blend because everyone suffers from different symptoms or a combination. Choose from the appropriate recipes below or combine the oils from other recipes if you need to. Begin using the formulas as soon as you feel the onset of PMT, for some it could be 3 days before their period, for others it could be as much as 7 to 10 days.

Essential oils for pre menstrual tension; Bergamot, Cedarwood, Chamomile (Roman), Clary Sage, Cypress, Fennel, Geranium, Grapefruit, Jasmine, Juniper, Lavender, Lemon, Marjoram, Neroli, Nutmeg, Patchouli, Peppermint, Rose, Ylang Ylang.

Carrier oils for pre menstrual tension; Sweet Almond, Coconut, Evening Primrose, Grapeseed, Olive.

❧ Massage Oils ❧

Blend all ingredients together and mix thoroughly. Massage in a clockwise motion around the abdomen and lower back, alternatively massage into the back of the neck and shoulders. Repeat daily for up to 14 days before menstruation begins. Leave to absorb into the skin, do not wash off. The following recipes will yield enough for 1 treatment.

Weeping/Low Moods Blend 1
2 tablespoons evening primrose oil
8 drops of bergamot
4 drops of grapefruit
2 drops of ylang ylang
1 drops of jasmine

Weeping/Low Moods Blend 2
2 tablespoons sweet almond oil
4 drops of grapefruit
4 drops of ylang ylang
3 drops of rose
3 drops of neroli
1 drop of bergamot

Bloating Blend 1

2 tablespoons evening primrose oil
6 drops of juniper
4 drops of carrot seed
2 drops of chamomile
2 drops of lemon
1 drop of peppermint

Irritability Blend 1

2 tablespoons grapeseed oil
4 drops of nutmeg
4 drops of geranium
4 drops of clary sage
3 drops of bergamot

Fatigue Blend 1

2 tablespoons sweet almond oil
6 drops of rosemary
6 drops of basil
3 drops of jasmine

Bloating Blend 2

2 tablespoons sweet almond oil
8 drops of clary sage
4 drops of fennel
2 drops of juniper
2 drops of peppermint

Irritability Blend 2

2 tablespoons coconut oil
6 drops of chamomile
3 drops of clary sage
3 drops of geranium
2 drops of bergamot
1 drop of lavender

Fatigue Blend 2

2 tablespoons coconut oil
4 drops of geranium
4 drops of fennel
4 drops of grapefruit
3 drops of bergamot

❧ Bath Oils ❧

Blend all ingredients together and mix thoroughly. Apply to the water after the bath has been filled. Agitate the water to disperse the oils around the bath. Soak for 20 minutes. The following recipes will yield enough for 1 treatment.

Weeping/Low Moods Blend 1

1 tablespoon sweet almond oil
7 drops of jasmine
3 drops of grapefruit

Weeping/Low Moods Blend 2

1 tablespoon grapeseed oil
3 drops of ylang ylang
3 drops of bergamot
2 drops of rosemary
1 drop of grapefruit
1 drop of jasmine

Irritability Blend 1

1 tablespoon grapeseed oil
6 drops of sandalwood
3 drops of neroli
3 drops of chamomile

Irritability Blend 2

1 tablespoon olive oil
5 drops of mandarin
5 drops of neroli
2 drops of lavender

❧ Body Mist ❧

Blend all ingredients together in a spray bottle and mix thoroughly. When needed, hold the bottle about 3 to 4 inches away from the body and spray liberally around the upper body. Repeat several times throughout the day. The following recipes will yield enough for approximately 2 days, depending on how often it is used.

Weeping/Low Moods Blend 1

50ml distilled water
10 drops of jasmine
5 drops of sandalwood
5 drops of ylang ylang
5 drops of lavender

Weeping/Low Moods Blend 2

50ml distilled water
10 drops of neroli
10 drops of ylang ylang
5 drops of grapefruit

Irritability Blend 1

50ml distilled water
10 drops of chamomile
10 drops of bergamot
5 drops of patchouli

Irritability Blend 2

50ml distilled water
10 drops of mandarin
10 drops of sandalwood
5 drops of neroli

Fatigue Blend 1

50ml distilled water
8 drops of rosemary
8 drops of clary sage
4 drops of rosemary
2 drops of basil
2 drops of peppermint

Fatigue Blend 2

50ml distilled water
10 drops of peppermint
5 drops of grapefruit
5 drops of rosemary
5 drops of jasmine

❧ Diffuser/Oil Burner ❧

Place water and essential oils at the top of the diffuser and light the candle below. Allow 10 to 15 minutes for the aroma to fill the room. The following blends should only be used during the day as some are designed to lift the spirits and may interfere with a good night's sleep.

Weeping/Low Moods Blend
4 drops of grapefruit
4 drops of bergamot

Irritability Blend
6 drops of mandarin
2 drops of neroli

Fatigue Blend
3 drops of rosemary
3 drops of basil
2 drops of peppermint

Psoriasis

Psoriasis is a common skin condition which occurs as a result of the over production of skin cells. It is characterized by red, scaly patches of skin that can become inflamed. It occurs most often on the torso, elbows, knees, feet and scalp, and tends to come and go sporadically. There is often an outbreak in times of stress (physical and emotional) and illness.

While steroid creams are often prescribed, the benefits of essential oils should not be overlooked. Many oils contain antiseptic, anti-inflammatory, antibacterial, antifungal, antiviral and skin soothing properties, making them an effective treatment for psoriasis.

Essential oils for psoriasis; Bergamot, Chamomile (Roman), Juniper, Lavender, Neroli, Patchouli, Sandalwood, Tea Tree.

Carrier oils for psoriasis; Apricot Kernel Oil, Avocado Oil, Borage Seed Oil, Coconut Oil, Evening Primrose Oil, Jojoba Oil.

❧ Treatment Oils ❧

Blend all ingredients together and apply to the affected area 3-4 times each day. Repeat daily until symptoms subside. The following recipes will yield enough for 1 day depending on the area being treated.

Blend 1
3 tablespoons avocado oil
4 drops of tea tree
4 drops of lavender
2 drops of neroli

Blend 2
3 tablespoons evening primrose oil
3 drops of sandalwood
3 drops of chamomile
3 drops of bergamot

Blend 3
3 tablespoons borage seed oil
10 drops of tea tree
2 drops of lavender

Blend 4
3 tablespoons jojoba oil
4 drops of juniper
2 drops of bergamot
2 drops of neroli
2 drops of lavender

❧ Treatment Moisturizers ❧

Blend all ingredients together and use immediately. Apply 3-4 times per day until symptoms subside. The following recipes will yield enough for 1 day depending on the area being treated.

Blend 1
2 tablespoons aloe vera gel
5 drops of tea tree
5 drops of lavender

Blend 2
2 tablespoons unscented moisturizer
10 drops of tea tree

❧ Treatment Baths ❧

If you are having an Epsom salt bath, add the salts first, followed by the water and then the essential oils. For a baking soda/dead sea salt bath, run the water first and add the soda/salts followed by the essential oils. Agitate the water to ensure the ingredients disperse.

Blend 1
½ cup baking soda
½ cup Dead Sea salts
1 tablespoons grapeseed oil
8 drops of chamomile
8 drops of patchouli
2 drops of lavender
2 drops of tea tree

Blend 2
1 cup Epsom salts
1 tablespoon coconut oil
15 drops tea tree

Blend 3
1 tablespoon olive oil
5 drops of neroli
5 drops of bergamot
5 drops of patchouli
5 drops of patchouli

Blend 4
1 cup Dead Sea salts
1 tablespoon olive oil
3 drops of chamomile
3 drops of juniper
3 drops of sandalwood
3 drops of lavender

❧ Treatment Shampoo for the Scalp ❧

Blend all ingredients in a jar or old shampoo bottle, mix thoroughly and apply to damp hair. Shake well before use. The following recipes will yield enough for 1 treatment.

Blend 1

5 tablespoons organic coconut milk
¼ cup liquid Castile soap
1 tablespoon evening primrose oil
1 tablespoon extra virgin olive oil
15 drops of tea tree
5 drops of chamomile

Blend 2

2 tablespoons apple cider vinegar
5 drops of patchouli
2 drops of sandalwood
2 drops of neroli

❧ Treatment Oils for the Scalp ❧

Blend all ingredients and massage thoroughly into the scalp using fingertips. Leave for 2-4 hours. Wash the hair using a chemical free shampoo or choose from one of the recipes above. Repeat 2-3 times per week. The following recipes will yield enough for 1 treatment on shoulder length hair.

Blend 1

½ cup warm extra virgin olive oil
15 drops of tea tree

Blend 2

½ cup apple cider vinegar
5 drops of chamomile
5 drops of juniper
5 drops of lavender

Rashes

Rashes can occur for a variety of reasons, both internal and external, and can be localized to one part of the body or they can affect larger areas. Allergic reactions, viral infections, bacterial infections, heat, or spicy food, etc. can all cause a rash to appear on the skin. Symptoms include blister formation, itching, small bumps on the skin, scaling, and skin discoloration. While essential oils can offer relief to some of these symptoms, it is always best to contact your doctor to discuss any potential underlying health issue.

Essential oils for rashes; Chamomile (Roman), Geranium, Lavender, Myrrh, Peppermint, Rose, Sandalwood.

Carrier oils for rashes; Coconut (Raw Virgin), Evening Primrose, Olive (Extra Virgin).

❧ Massage Oils ❧

Blend all ingredients together and mix thoroughly. Massage the formula directly over the affected area and leave the oils to absorb into the skin. Repeat 2 to 3 times per day as and when is needed. Stop the treatment as soon as the skin normalizes. The following recipes will yield enough for 1 treatment on a specific area. You will need to increase the ingredients if massaging over the entire body – use 3 tablespoons of carrier oil blended with 15 drops of essential oils.

Blend 1
1 tablespoon coconut oil (raw virgin)
8 drops of lavender
2 drops of chamomile

Blend 2
1 tablespoon olive oil (extra virgin)
5 drops of chamomile
4 drops of peppermint
1 drop of tea tree

Blend 3
1 tablespoon coconut oil (raw virgin)
4 drops of geranium
3 drops of sandalwood

Blend 4
1 tablespoon olive oil (extra virgin)
6 drops of myrrh
4 drops of lavender

❧ Bath Oils ❧

Blend all ingredients together and mix thoroughly. Fill the bath with warm water (not hot), and once filled, add the essential oil blend. Agitate the water to disperse the oils and soak for 15 minutes.

Blend 1
1 tablespoon olive oil
5 drops of lavender
5 drops of chamomile

Blend 2
1 tablespoon olive oil
5 drops of myrrh
3 drops of peppermint
2 drops of chamomile

❧ Body Mist ❧

A body mist can be used as an alternative to a massage blend, particularly if you are out of the house during the day. Always use fractionated coconut oil in your blends as this particular type of coconut oil does not solidify in cool temperatures. Blend all ingredients together in a spray bottle and shake well to mix. Spray the area affected several times throughout the day. The following recipes will yield enough for approximately 2 days, depending on the size of the area being treated.

Blend 1
50ml coconut oil
10 drops of chamomile
4 drops of peppermint
1 drop of geranium

Blend 2
50ml coconut oil
8 drops of lavender
7 drops of myrrh

❧ Cold Compress ❧

Prepare a bowl of cold water and add your chosen essential oils. Place the compress into the water to soak for 2 minutes. Remove and wring out any excess water. Apply over the affected area and leave for 1 hour. Each time the compress starts to warm to body heat, dip back into the water to refresh and apply again.

Blend 1
6 drops of lavender

Blend 2
3 drops of chamomile
3 drops of peppermint

Rheumatism

Rheumatism is a general term that indicates any of the various diseases associated with the musculoskeletal system, involving pain in the muscles and stiffness in the joints. However, rheumatism is essentially a disorder in which pain is experienced in the muscles and soft tissue as opposed to arthritis, where pain and stiffness is associated with the joints. Rheumatism, also referred to as fibrositis, normally only affects one group of muscles at a time, and can be the result of a cold or chill, injury to a muscle, ligament or tendon, or repetitive strain where the constant use of one particular group of muscles causes them to become weakened and painful.

Essential oils for rheumatism; Chamomile (Roman), Cypress, Ginger, Juniper, Lavender, Marjoram, Peppermint, Rosemary, Thyme.

Carrier oils for rheumatism; Avocado, Coconut, Grapeseed, Olive, Sesame.

❧ Massage Oils ❧

Blend all ingredients together and mix thoroughly. Massage the formula into the affected area twice daily, once in the morning and again at night. Leave the oils to absorb into the skin, do not wash off. Skip a day every 2 days as the essential oils will have enough residual effects so they don't have to be used every day. The following recipes will yield enough for 1 treatment on a specific area. You may need to increase the amount used a larger area, or if more than 1 area is being treated, for example, both legs.

Blend 1
1 tablespoon grapeseed oil
6 drops of rosemary
3 drops of lavender
1 drop of peppermint

Blend 2
1 tablespoon sesame oil
3 drops of marjoram
3 drops of juniper
3 drops of eucalyptus
1 drop of ginger

Blend 3
1 tablespoon melted coconut oil
3 drops of lavender
3 drops of rosemary
3 drops of cypress
1 drop of peppermint

Blend 4
1 tablespoon olive oil
5 drops of juniper
5 drops of lavender

❧ Bath Oils ❧

Blend and mix the ingredients together. Fill the bath with hot water and once filled, add your chosen blend. Agitate the water to disperse the oils, and soak for 20 minutes. If you are using Epsom salts, always add the salts before running the water.

Blend 1

1 tablespoon olive oil
6 drops of chamomile
6 drops of rosemary
3 drops of peppermint

Blend 2

1 tablespoon grapeseed oil
5 drops of marjoram
5 drops of juniper
4 drops of lavender
1 drop of ginger

Blend 3

1 tablespoon avocado oil
8 drops of lavender
6 drops of peppermint
1 drop of thyme

Blend 4

1 tablespoon grapeseed oil
4 drops of rosemary
4 drops of cypress
3 drops of juniper
3 drops of lavender
1 drop of ginger

Shingles

Shingles, also known as herpes zoster, is a viral infection caused by the same virus that causes chicken pox. It most commonly attacks adults between the ages of 40 and 70, although it can frequently occur in other age groups, especially at times of stress or when a person becomes physically run down. It is a painful, distressing condition where the rash develops from reddened raised areas into blisters that join together and rapidly rupture and crust. The rash typically progresses in a band around one side of the chest, trunk or abdomen. The main complaint following an attack of shingles is the actual pain experience and as such, essential oils that provide pain relief should be used.

Essential oils for shingles; Bergamot, Chamomile (Roman), Eucalyptus, Lavender, Lemon, Peppermint, Sandalwood, Tea Tree.

Carrier oils for shingles; Fractionated Coconut Oil and Raw Virgin Coconut Oil.

❧ Massage Oils ❧

Blend all ingredients together and mix thoroughly. Gently massage the formula into the affected area each day, first thing in the morning. The following recipes will yield enough for 1 treatment. In some instances the skin may be too sensitive to touch, in which case a body spray is recommended (recipes below).

Blend 1
1 tablespoon melted coconut oil (raw, virgin)
4 drops of peppermint
4 drops of lavender
2 drops of bergamot

Blend 2
1 tablespoon melted coconut oil
5 drops of eucalyptus
2 drops of bergamot
2 drops of lavender
1 drop of tea tree

Blend 3
1 tablespoon melted coconut oil (raw, virgin)
4 drops of lavender
4 drops of chamomile
2 drops of tea tree

Blend 4
1 tablespoon melted coconut oil
5 drops of chamomile
3 drops of lavender
2 drops of thyme

❧ Body Spray ❧

Fractionated coconut oil is recommended for use in a spray bottle for the treatment of shingles as coconut oil is light, easily absorbed by the skin, nourishing and has excellent healing properties. Raw Virgin Coconut Oil should not be used as this will have to be melted, and may possibly solidify in the bottle if left in a cool place. Blend all ingredients together in a spray bottle and shake well to mix. Apply to the affected area daily. Do not exceed 3 daily applications. The following recipes will yield enough for 3 treatments (1 day).

Blend 1

3 tablespoons coconut oil
10 drops of chamomile
8 drops of lavender
2 drops of tea tree

Blend 2

3 tablespoons coconut oil
8 drops of tea tree
6 drops of peppermint
4 drops of bergamot
2 drops of chamomile

Blend 3

3 tablespoons coconut oil
5 drops of lemon
5 drops of tea tree
5 drops of eucalyptus
5 drops of lavender

Blend 4

3 tablespoons coconut oil
10 drops of peppermint
5 drops of lavender
3 drops of chamomile
2 drops of lemon

Sinusitis

The sinuses are cavities in the bones of the face and skull, and are lined with mucus membrane similar to that lining the nose. As the openings from the nose into the sinuses are very narrow, they quickly become blocked when the mucus membrane of the nose becomes swollen during a cold, hay fever or catarrh, resulting in the infection becoming trapped inside the sinus. The classical signs of sinusitis include pain and tenderness in the relevant areas of the face and head, frequently accompanied by a thick nasal discharge. In acute attacks, head and facial pain can be severe and the sufferer may feel quite ill, sometimes experiencing a high temperature.

Essential oils for sinusitis; Basil, Eucalyptus, Juniper, Lavender, Lemon, Peppermint, Pine, Rosemary, Tea Tree, Thyme.

Carrier oils for sinusitis; Sweet Almond, Coconut, Jojoba.

❧ Massage Oils ❧

Blend all ingredients together and mix thoroughly. Gently massage the formula around the nose, cheeks, forehead, behind the ears, and front and back of the neck. Apply the blend twice per day. The following recipes will yield enough for 1 day (2 treatments).

Blend 1
3 tablespoons sweet almond
8 drops of rosemary
4 drops of peppermint
3 drops of thyme

Blend 2
3 tablespoons jojoba oil
10 drops of eucalyptus
3 drops of rosemary
1 drop of pine
1 drop of basil

Blend 3
3 tablespoons coconut oil
5 drops of geranium
5 drops of eucalyptus
4 drops of peppermint
1 drop of lavender

Blend 4
3 tablespoons sweet almond oil
6 drops of lemon
6 drops of peppermint
2 drops of juniper
1 drop of tea tree

Inhalation

Prepare a bowl of steaming hot water, add your chosen essential oils, cover your head with a towel, close your eyes, and inhale the aroma of the oils for 2 to 3 minutes. Repeat once or twice per day as and when is needed.

Blend 1

3 drops of lavender
2 drops of peppermint
1 drop of tea tree

Blend 2

4 drops of eucalyptus
1 drop of lemon
1 drop of pine

Snoring

Snoring can not only disrupt sleep but it can also have adverse effects on health and possibly relationships, so finding an effective treatment is very important. Certain essential oils help relieve snoring as they work on clearing nasal passageways and reduce any inflammation around nasal openings.

Essential oils for snoring; Basil, Cedarwood, Chamomile, Cypress, Eucalyptus, Lavender, Marjoram, Peppermint, Sandalwood, Thyme.

Carrier oils for snoring; Sweet Almond, Coconut, Olive.

❧ Massage Oils ❧

Blend all ingredients and mix thoroughly. Massage the formula into the front of the neck, upper chest, tops of shoulders and back of the neck. Apply each night before bedtime. The following recipes will make 1 treatment.

Blend 1
1 tablespoon olive oil
3 drops of marjoram
3 drops of thyme
3 drops chamomile
1 drop of lavender

Blend 2
1 tablespoon sweet almond
4 drops of sandalwood
2 drops of geranium
2 drops of cedarwood
2 drops of eucalyptus

Blend 3
1 tablespoon coconut oil
5 drops of lavender
5 drops of marjoram

Blend 4
1 tablespoon sweet almond oil
3 drops of peppermint
3 drops of lemon
1 drop of lavender

❧ Pillow Mist ❧

Blend all ingredients in a spray bottle and mix thoroughly. Hold the bottle about 3 – 4 inches away from the pillow and spray liberally. Repeat each night before bedtime. The following recipes will make treatments for 3 to 4 nights.

Blend 1

30ml distilled water
20 drops of marjoram
5 drops of lavender
5 drops of peppermint

Blend 2

30ml lavender hydrosol
10 drops of lavender
10 drops of sandalwood
10 drops of chamomile

Blend 3

30ml distilled water
15 drops of eucalyptus
10 drops of marjoram
5 drops of lemon

Blend 4

30ml distilled water
10 drops of peppermint
5 drops of thyme
5 drops of sandalwood
5 drops of lavender
3 drops of chamomile
2 drops of cedarwood

Stress

Stress is any factor that causes an emotional or mental strain on the body, largely caused by worry over financial problems, work load, future circumstances and/or relationships. People have different ways of reacting to stress, some will see a particular situation as being very stressful while others may be able to deal with it in a more calm and logical manner. Common symptoms of stress include racing heart or palpitations, sleeping problems, loss of appetite, sweating and difficulty concentrating. It has been estimated that stress is the underlying cause of 75% of disease, and as a result, should be managed in an appropriate way.

Essential oils help to bring the body back into balance by promoting relaxation, easing anxiety, stabilizing breathing, and creating a calmness in both body and mind.

Essential oils for stress; Bergamot, Cedarwood, Chamomile (Roman), Clary Sage, Frankincense, Geranium, Jasmine, Juniper, Lavender, Marjoram, Melissa, Neroli, Orange, Petitgrain, Rose, Rosewood, Sandalwood, Valerian, Ylang Ylang,

Carrier oils for stress; Sweet Almond, Avocado, Borage Seed, Coconut, Evening Primrose, Grapeseed, Hazelnut, Jojoba, Olive, Sesame.

❧ Bath Oils ❧

Bathing with essential oils is one of the most relaxing ways to unwind from any stressful situation. Simple add your chosen oils to a carrier oil, shake to combine ingredients and add to the bath water. Swirl the oils around in the bath to disperse. Soak for 20 – 30 minutes.

Blend 1
1 tablespoon avocado oil
8 drops of lavender

Blend 2
1 tablespoon jojoba oil
4 drops of bergamot
4 drops of chamomile

Blend 3
1 tablespoon sweet almond oil
4 drops of clary sage
3 drops of marjoram

Blend 4
1 tablespoon evening primrose oil
2 drops of sandalwood
2 drops of ylang ylang
2 drops of chamomile
1 drop of lavender

❧ Massage Oils ❧

Massaging essential oils into the skin is a wonderful way to relax both the body and mind, and can be used effectively to treat stress. Blend all ingredients and massage the formula into the upper chest, across the shoulders, back of the neck and any other tense areas. Repeat as often as is needed. The following recipes will yield enough for 1 treatment.

Blend 1
2 tablespoons jojoba oil
5 drops of rosewood
5 drops of chamomile
2 drops of lavender
2 drops of marjoram

Blend 2
2 tablespoons sweet almond oil
5 drops of frankincense
4 drops of rosewood
4 drops of lavender

Blend 3
2 tablespoons apricot kernel oil
6 drops of marjoram
2 drops of petitgrain
2 drops of chamomile
2 drops of melissa

Blend 4
2 tablespoons grapeseed oil
4 drops of lavender
4 drops of jasmine
2 drops of rosewood
2 drops of sandalwood
2 drops of chamomile

❧ Bath Salts ❧

Bath salts have the same benefits as bath oils, however they have additional detoxification properties due to the added ingredient of salt. If you are adding Epsom salts to a bath, put this ingredient in before you fill the bath, then add the essential oils to the water. If, on the other hand, you are adding Dead Sea salt, this can go in together with the essential oils after the bath has been filled. Swirl the formula around the water to disperse the oils and salt.

Blend 1
2 cups Dead Sea salt
1 tablespoon avocado oil
10 drops of lavender
10 drops of clary sage
8 drops of sandalwood

Blend 2
1 cup Epsom salt
½ cup baking soda
1 tablespoon olive oil
5 drops of marjoram
5 drops of chamomile
5 drops of grapefruit

Blend 3
1½ cups Epsom salts
1 tablespoon evening primrose oil
10 drops of bergamot
5 drops of juniper
5 drops of chamomile
5 drops of lavender

Blend 4
2 cups Dead Sea salts
1 tablespoon olive oil
8 drops of frankincense
8 drops of bergamot
8 drops of clary sage

Diffuser/Oil Burner ❧

To use this method, simply fill the bowl at the top of the burner with water, followed by your chosen essential oils. Then place a lighted tea lighted underneath the bowl. Allow the relaxing aromas of the essential oils to fill the room.

Blend 1
10 drops of lavender

Blend 2
5 drops of frankincense
5 drops of jasmine

Blend 3
5 drops of clary sage
5 drops of bergamot

Blend 4
10 drops of chamomile

❧ Mist Sprays ❧

An aromatherapy spritzer/mist spray can be misted lightly on the face, neck or body throughout the day to help lessen feelings of anxiety. Simply place the distilled water or hydrosol and essential oils in a spray bottle, shake well and mist liberally. Always hold the bottle about 3 to 4 inches away from the area being sprayed.

Blend 1
50ml distilled water
10 drops of bergamot
10 drops of lavender
5 drops of frankincense

Blend 2
50ml distilled water
15 drops of clary sage
10 drops of lavender
8 drops of lemon

Blend 3

50ml lavender hydrosol
10 drops of grapefruit
10 drops of ylang ylang
8 drops of jasmine

Blend 4

50ml distilled water
10 drops of patchouli
10 drops of orange (sweet)
10 drops of cypress

Sunburn

Sunburn is classified as a first degree burn as it only affects the outer skin, and as a result, can be effectively treated using essential oils.

Essential oils for sunburn; Chamomile, Geranium, Lavender, Peppermint, Tea Tree.

Essential oils for sunburn; Sweet Almond Oil, Avocado, Coconut, Aloe Vera Gel (not a carrier oil but a valuable treatment for sunburn).

❧ Treatment Oils ❧

Blend all ingredients together and mix thoroughly. Apply to the affected area 3-4 times per day. The following recipes will yield enough for 1 day.

Blend 1
2 tablespoons aloe vera gel
6 drops of lavender
6 drops of chamomile

Blend 2
2 tablespoons aloe vera gel
12 drops of lavender

Blend 3
2 tablespoons coconut oil
8 drops of lavender
4 drops of peppermint

Blend 4
2 tablespoons avocado oil
4 drops of chamomile
4 drops of geranium
4 drops of tea tree

❧ Treatment Spritz ❧

Blend all ingredients together in a spray bottle and mix well. Keep refrigerated and use several times a day on the area of sunburn. Shake well before use. The following recipes will last approximately 2 days.

Blend 1
50ml distilled water
1 teaspoon aloe vera juice
4 drops of lavender
4 drops of chamomile

Blend 2
50 ml distilled water
1 tablespoon aloe vera juice
10 drops of tea tree

Blend 3
50ml distilled water
15 drops of lavender

Blend 4
50ml distilled water
2 tablespoons aloe vera juice
4 drops of lavender
4 drops of peppermint

Travel Sickness

Travel or motion sickness is a very common complaint and can occur while in a car, or on a plane, boat or train. Common symptoms include nausea, vomiting, dizziness, cold sweats, and sometimes hot sweats. It is a very miserable experience for sufferers but thankfully essential oils can help to ease, and sometimes, alleviate symptoms.

Essential oils for travel sickness; Chamomile (Roman), Frankincense, Ginger, Peppermint.

Carrier oils for travel sickness; Fractionated Coconut Oil.

❧ Massage Oils ❧

Blend ingredients together and mix thoroughly. Massage the formula on the abdomen just before travel. Massage using circular, clockwise movements. The following recipes will yield enough for 1 treatment.

Blend 1
1 tablespoon coconut oil
4 drops of peppermint
2 drops of frankincense

Blend 2
1 tablespoon coconut oil
3 drops of chamomile
2 drops of peppermint
1 drop of ginger

Varicose Veins

Varicose veins are the result of poor blood circulation in the leg area. Prolonged periods of sitting or standing, pregnancy, obesity or wearing tight clothing can inhibit circulation resulting in veins becoming weakened and stretched. These weakened veins become larger and twisted, and can be seen clearly through the skin. The use of essential oils can be very beneficial with this condition, helping to improve circulation and reduce the appearance of varicose veins.

Essential oils for varicose veins; Cypress, Geranium, Grapefruit, Lavender, Lemon, Lemongrass, Peppermint.

Carrier oils for varicose veins; Sweet Almond, Coconut, Evening Primrose, Extra Virgin Olive Oil.

❧ Massage Oils ❧

Blend ingredients together and mix thoroughly. Gently apply the blend to the bottom of the vein and massage upwards towards the heart with light pressure. Do this for approximately 4 – 5 minutes. Repeat twice daily, both morning and night. With consistent application, results should be seen after 1 to 2 months. The following recipes will yield enough for 1 day (2 treatments).

Blend 1
2 tablespoons melted raw virgin coconut oil
15 drops of cypress
10 drops of lemon
5 drops of lavender

Blend 2
2 tablespoons sweet almond oil
30 drops of cypress

Blend 3
2 tablespoons raw virgin coconut oil
1 tablespoon evening primrose oil
10 drops of lavender
10 drops of grapefruit
5 drops of cypress
5 drops of lemongrass

Blend 4
2 tablespoons sweet almond oil
20 drops of cypress
5 drops of geranium
5 drops of peppermint

12
Aromatherapy for the Home

❧ Air Freshener ❧

Fill a bowl of boiling water and add your chosen essential oils. Place on a secure counter in any room, e.g. kitchen, bathroom, bedroom, and leave to rest. The beautiful aroma will fill the room in about 10 minutes. The recipe below is a beautiful combination but you can use any of your favorite oils.

Air Freshener Blend
5 drops of jasmine
3 drops of neroli

❧ Bathroom Cleaner ❧

Blend all ingredients together in a spray bottle and mix thoroughly. The essential oils used in these recipes have fantastic antibacterial properties, and are a great alternative to harsh chemical cleaners you can buy in the store. The following recipe should last approximately 2 weeks, depending on the number of bathrooms you have. Shake well each time before use.

Bathroom Cleaner
1 cup distilled water
2 tablespoons baking soda
4 tablespoons liquid castile soap
10 drops of lemon
5 drops of peppermint
5 drops of tea tree

❧ Bed Bugs ❧

Bed bugs are small, parasitic insects that are nocturnal and survive by living on human blood. They are attracted to the warmth so typically inhabit bedding and sleeping areas. Certain essential oils are an effective way to get rid of these pesky creatures.

Blend all ingredients in a spray bottle and shake well to mix. Strip the bedding and spray the mattress, leave to breathe for several hours. Diffuse the room while the mattress is bare. Wash the linens and place 3 drops of lemon essential oil to the fabric conditioner in the washer/dryer. When the bed has been made up, continue to use the spray on the pillow cases and sheets once every day. In between linen changes, spray the mattress again, leave to breathe and diffuse the room. The following recipes for the spray should last for 3 to 4 days on 1 bed.

Spray Blend
1 cup distilled water
15 drops of lemon
5 drops of peppermint

Diffuse Blend
3 drops of lemongrass
2 drops of lavender
1 drop of clove

❧ Carpet Cleaner ❧

Add the essential oils to the baking soda and blend well using a plastic or wooden spoon. Make sure to break up all the clumps. To use, lightly shake the mixture evenly over the carpet or rug, and leave to infuse for 2 to 3 hours. Vacuum, and you will have clean, fresh smelling carpets throughout your home.

Carpet Cleaner Blend
1 cup baking soda
10 drops of lavender

❧ Disinfecting Spray ❧

Blend all ingredients together in a spray bottle and mix thoroughly. This is an excellent substitute for chemical cleaners and can be used on all surfaces in the house. When sprayed, leave on for 10 seconds and wipe off with a cloth or paper towel. The following recipes will yield enough for approximately 1 week depending on how often it is used.

Blend 1
1 cup of distilled water
¼ cup apple cider vinegar
15 drops of lemon
10 drops of tea tree
5 drops of grapefruit

Blend 2
1 cup of distilled water
¼ cup apple cider vinegar
10 cups of lavender
10 drops of lavender
10 drops of peppermint

❧ Floor Cleaner ❧

Fill a bucket or basin with lukewarm water, add ¼ cup of apple cider vinegar and your chosen essential oils. Wipe with a floor mop or cloth.

Tile Floor Blend
10 drops of lemon
5 drops of eucalyptus

Wooden Floor Blend
10 drops of orange
5 drops of lavender

❧ Furniture Polish ❧

Blend all ingredients together in a spray bottle and shake well to mix. Spray onto furniture and polish off with a clean, soft cloth. The jojoba and olive oils moisturize the wood, while the essential oils will leave a beautiful shine. The following recipes should be used within 1 month.

Blend 1
½ cup jojoba oil
¼ cup white vinegar
20 drops of lemon

Blend 2
½ cup olive oil
¼ cup white vinegar
15 drops of orange
5 drops of lavender

❧ Insect Repellent ❧

Insect repellents made with essential oils are a more natural and safer alternative to products you can buy in the store. Blend all the ingredients together and mix thoroughly. Massage the formula into exposed areas of skin, for example the ankles or shoulders. Due to photosensitivity, only use the following recipes in the evening, do not use when exposed to sun. The following recipes will yield enough for 1 treatment.

Massage Blend 1
1 tablespoon grapeseed oil
5 drops of lemongrass
3 drops of geranium

Massage Blend 2
1 tablespoon grapeseed oil
4 drops of lemon
2 drops of basil
2 drops of peppermint

Bug sprays and diffusing essential oils are also effective ways to deter insects. For bug spray, diffuse all ingredients in a spray bottle and shake well to mix. Spray onto exposed areas of skin. Do not use in the sun. Shake well before use. Use the diffuser in the evening when at home, safely place on top of a table or below it.

Spray Blend
1 cup distilled water
15 drops of lemongrass
5 drops of eucalyptus

Diffuse Blend
5 drops of lemon
1 drop of lavender

❧ Laundry ❧

Add 3 drops of lemon or jasmine oil to the fabric conditioner section in your washing machine. The aroma of these oils will infuse into your clothes, creating a beautiful, fresh scent.

❧ Room Spray/Linen Spray ❧

Fill a spray bottle with water (preferably distilled or filtered), and add essential oils. Shake well before use. Spray onto clothes or throughout the room when you want to create a beautiful, fresh aroma.

Calming Room Spray
15 drops of lavender
15 drops of chamomile
15 drops of rosemary

Uplifting Room Spray
15 drops of geranium
15 drops of lemon
15 drops of ylang ylang

❧ Vacuum Cleaner ❧

Add 3 drops of orange or lavender oil to the filter of your vacuum. If there is no filter, add the drops of essential oils onto a cotton ball and place in the disposable bag. Each time you vacuum the scent will infuse into the room.

❧ Waste Bins ❧

Place a paper towel or tissue at the bottom of your bin. Add 4 to 5 drops of essential oil onto the towel or tissue, and allow the oils to keep your bin fresh and germ free. Choose from lavender, orange, lemon, pine, lemongrass or tea tree.

❧ Window or Glass Cleaner ❧

Combine all ingredients in a spray bottle, shake well to mix, spray onto your window or glass surface, and remove using a microfiber cloth or newspaper.

Window/Glass Cleaner Blend
1 cup distilled water
½ cup white vinegar
8 drops of lavender
7 drops of orange

48288157R00120

Made in the USA
Lexington, KY
23 December 2015